Pain

Creative Approaches to Effective Management

Also by Eloise C. J. Carr and Eileen M. Mann:

Partnering Patients to Manage Pain After Surgery (video and 48-page booklet) Institute of Health and Community Studies, Bournemouth University, 1998.

Pain

Creative Approaches to Effective Management

ELOISE C. J. CARR
and
EILEEN M. MANN

(in association with the Institute of Health and Community
Studies, Bournemouth University)

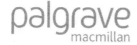
palgrave
macmillan

Published by
PALGRAVE MACMILLAN
Houndmills, Basingstoke, Hampshire RG21 6XS and
175 Fifth Avenue, New York, N.Y. 10010
Companies and representatives throughout the world

PALGRAVE MACMILLAN is the global academic imprint of the Palgrave Macmillan division of St. Martin's Press, LLC and of Palgrave Macmillan Ltd. Macmillan® is a registered trademark in the United States, United Kingdom and other countries. Palgrave is a registered trademark in the European Union and other countries.

ISBN 0–333–77639–9 paperback

This book is printed on paper suitable for recycling and made from fully managed and sustained forest sources.

A catalogue record for this book is available from the British Library.

Editing and origination by Aardvark Editorial, Mendham, Suffolk

10 9 8 7 6 5 4
09 08 07 06 05 04 03

Printed and bound in Great Britain by
Creative Print & Design (Wales), Ebbw Vale

Contents

List of figures ix

List of tables x

Preface xi

Introduction xii

Acknowledgements xiv

1   The multidimensional nature of pain 1
Learning outcomes 1
Indicative reading 1
Background 2
Why has pain been so misunderstood? 2
An introduction to neurophysiology 5
Gate Control Theory in understanding the complexity
   of pain 17
Why can pain get worse when the damage appears to be
   healing? 20
Addiction, tolerance and dependence 22
Conclusion 24
Suggested further reading 25
Multiple-choice questionnaire 26
Answers for the multiple-choice questionnaire 27
Glossary of terms 28

2   Assessing pain 30
Learning outcomes 30
Indicative reading 30
Background 31
Why assess pain? 31
When to assess pain 32
How to assess pain 33
Nurse factors affecting the assessment of pain 35
Patient factors affecting the assessment of pain 36

Pain assessment scales   38
Changing practice – introducing a pain assessment tool   44
Conclusion   46
Suggested further reading   46
Multiple-choice questionnaire   47
Answers for the multiple-choice questionnaire   49

3 **Managing acute pain**   **51**
   Learning outcomes   51
   Indicative reading   51
   Background   52
   The patients' perspective – experiencing acute pain   52
   What are acute pain services?   54
   The future of acute pain services   56
   Pharmacological approaches to pain management   57
   Non-pharmacological approaches to acute
      pain management   72
   Conclusion   77
   Suggested further reading   77
   Multiple-choice questionnaire   78
   Answers for the multiple-choice questionnaire   80

4 **Managing chronic pain**   **81**
   Learning outcomes   81
   Indicative reading   81
   Background   82
   What is chronic non-malignant pain?   83
   The patient's perspective – experiencing chronic pain   83
   Managing chronic pain   85
   Pharmacological approaches to pain management   87
   Regional nerve blocks   91
   Non-pharmacological strategies for managing chronic pain   92
   Physical techniques for managing pain   92
   Psychological interventions   97
   Trusting therapeutic relationships   100
   Social activities   100
   Exercise   101
   Professional collaboration in pain management   102
   Chronic pain clinics   102
   Conclusion   104
   Suggested further reading   105
   Multiple-choice questionnaire   106
   Answers for the multiple-choice questionnaire   107

**5   Recognising the barriers to effective
      pain relief**   **109**
      Learning outcomes   109
      Indicative reading   109
      Background   109
      Health care professionals   110
      Improving practice   113
      Patient barriers to effective pain management   115
      Organisational aspects   119
      Work demands in the clinical area   119
      Limitations of prescribing   123
      Interprofessional pain education   123
      Improving practice   124
      Conclusion   125
      Suggested further reading   126
      Multiple-choice questionnaire   126
      Answers for the multiple-choice questionnaire   128

6   Managing pain in vulnerable patients   **130**
      Learning outcomes   130
      Indicative reading   130
      Background   131
      Defining the barriers   133
      Pain in the elderly   134
      Pain management in the cognitively impaired
        elderly patient   135
      Learning disability and brain-injured patients   141
      Neonates and preverbal children   141
      Ethnic minorities   148
      Conclusion   150
      Suggested further reading   151
      Multiple-choice questionnaire   152
      Answers for the multiple-choice questionnaire   154

7   Nursing patients with challenging pain   **156**
      Learning outcomes   156
      Indicative reading   156
      Background   157
      Pain following a serious burn   159
      Pain in the patient with a spinal injury   162
      Pain in patients with sickle-cell disease   164
      Mood disorder and pain   166
      Substance abuse   169

Intractable pain and secondary gain   175
Conclusion   180
Suggested further reading   180
Multiple-choice questionnaire   181
Answers for the multiple-choice questionnaire   183

References   185

Index   198

List of figures

1.1 The synaptic activity of A delta fibres in the spinal cord   6
1.2 The synaptic activity of C fibres in the spinal cord   9
1.3 Activity of A beta fibres in the spinal cord   10
1.4 Touch, pinprick and burning pain sensations transmitted
     to the brain via the dorsal horn of the spinal cord   10
1.5 Gate Control Theory – how a gate may be opened
     or closed   11
1.6 Response to the 'chemical cascade' caused by
     tissue damage   14
1.7 Receptor activity   17

2.1 Visual analogue scale   39
2.2 Examples of pain scales   40
2.3 London Hospital Pain Chart   40
2.4 Short-form McGill Pain Questionnaire (SF-MPQ)   42
2.5 Chart for recording acute pain intensity   43

3.1 Entonox delivery apparatus   66
3.2 World Health Organization pain ladder   68
3.3 Location of the needle in the epidural space through
     which a catheter is threaded to enable continuous
     drug administration   72
3.4 A TENS machine attached to a patient's belt with the
     electrodes applied to the right side of his back   73

4.1 Acupuncture/acupressure point for nausea/PONV   94

6.1 Behaviours that help to indicate pain   138
6.2 Behaviours rated on the Liverpool Infant Distress Score   143
6.3 Score for facial expression   144
6.4 CHEOPS assessment categories   145

7.1 Physical and psychosocial influences on pain   158

List of tables

1.1   Activity of opioids at the three receptor sites   16

6.1   Matrix for identifying barriers to effective pain
      management   133
6.2   Types of disease and potential pain   137
6.3   CRIES pain assessment tool   144

Preface

Research documenting the undertreatment of pain can be found with regularity in the health care literature of the past 30 years. Advances in pain control have bought improvements for certain groups, but overall the problem of inadequate pain management persists across age groups, cultures, hospitals and the community.

The 'knowledge deficit' is acknowledged to be the most frequent reason for inadequate pain management, and education is probably the most important tool available to counteract this. Yet pain education is often neglected when attempting to squeeze all those other important subjects into the pre-registration curriculum, despite pain being one of the main reasons people consult their general practitioners and an experience that so often accompanies any interaction with the health care services.

These challenges can be targets for our educational initiatives, but a question remains: how can education change practice? We set out, a few years ago, to deliver some pain units to experienced nurses working across a range of clinical areas. In our teaching, we included small exercises encouraging them to collect information from their own clinical area and then reflect on these findings along with those from research studies. The impact of bringing those two dimensions together was tremendous. Suddenly, there was an energy, created by the tension between what was happening in practice and what *might* happen in practice – the possibility – a vision. Bridging the disordered world of practice endorsed our student-centered approach in tackling pain education and, as they say, 'We haven't looked back.'

We hope that you will enjoy this book and feel that we share with your struggles and frustrations; more importantly, however, we hope that it gives you the confidence to use the knowledge you have gleaned to provide the best possible care for those who suffer in pain.

ELOISE C. J. CARR
EILEEN M. MANN

Introduction

HOW THIS BOOK IS ORGANISED

This textbook has been structured around seven key chapters, starting with the multidimensional nature of pain. It is important to work through this chapter first as it forms the basis of the learning that follows. Before any strategies can be implemented to reduce pain, it is imperative that pain is carefully assessed as this forms the baseline for evaluation. Assessment is the linchpin of effective pain management, and we urge you to work through Chapter 2 after Chapter 1. You may then choose either acute or chronic pain, whichever is most appropriate to your own learning and interest. Barriers to effective pain management will make you want to implement change, and we suggest that you read the relevant chapter once you are armed with the knowledge from previous chapters. Finally, the last two chapters take a pragmatic view of how to manage pain with people who are vulnerable or whose pain is challenging. With the exception of children and the elderly, many of these groups do not receive regular mention in pain textbooks. We have tried to provide realistic approaches and further reading to help you.

HOW TO USE THIS BOOK

We suggest that you first buy an A4 ring-binder, seven section dividers (one for each chapter) and a nice thick pad of A4 paper. As you work through each chapter, you can thus make notes and file them; it is also useful to have somewhere to put any references you follow up.

Each chapter begins with several learning outcomes. These are the goals of learning and you should, by the end of each chapter, be able to achieve them. We include some indicative reading to give you some background and understanding before you start the chapter.

Scattered through each chapter are a number of different features, as outlined below:

- *Activities:* Within the text are activities for you to complete, based on what you have just been reading. These are central to your learning and we strongly urge you to take some time to complete them. They will give you a much greater insight and understanding of the topic being discussed.

- *Time out:* These sections are designed to provide some 'thinking' time and a bit of space to jot down reflections on personal experience. They can be undertaken on your own, or better still with a colleague. We can learn much from the experience of others, and working together may help to open up discussion.

- *Case histories:* These are illustrations, usually from our own practice, that relate the experience of a person/family and their pain. There are usually some questions for you to reflect on at the end.

- *'Coffee break':* It is important for you to have a break, so we have taken the liberty of providing you with an excuse.

Where possible, we have also included diagrams to simplify the text. Factual information may be listed and placed in boxes for clarity and quick reference.

At the end of each chapter is a further reading list, the references cited in each chapter appearing at the end of the book. It has not been our intention that you read everything but that you 'cherry pick' any items that will inform your own interests. We have tried to direct you to chapters and articles that are both informative and well written.

HOW CAN I ASSESS MY OWN LEARNING?

This is not a standard question, but we feel that it is helpful to gain some feedback on the work you have completed. At the end of each chapter are 10 multiple-choice questions. Try to complete them before referring to the answers provided as they are a quick and simple way of assessing your understanding. If you are a registered nurse, remember that this work can contribute to your portfolio and will be useful evidence that you are fulfilling the requirements of PREP and keeping clinically up to date. We hope, too, that your study will be an enjoyable experience.

Acknowledgements

We thank the NHS Executive South and West, who funded a teacher project to help us to develop open learning materials in pain management.

It is with gratitude that we acknowledge the contribution of Lynne Humphreys at the Institute of Health and Community Studies, Bournemouth University, who expertly (and in her own time) painstakingly read our manuscript for corrections.

Our own students shared our desire to improve pain management and enthusiastically used our novel approaches to learning; we are grateful to them for describing to us their experience.

Richenda Milton-Thompson has been totally committed in her belief in our ability to write a book, and we thank her for her constant supply of encouragement. Susan Merner at Poole Hospital (NHS) Trust library has never flinched at a constant request for books and articles and deserves our thanks.

With any endeavour of this sort, it is always our families to whom we owe so much. It is with genuine gratitude that we thank Tim and Peter for their selfless support, understanding and technical wizardry on the computer.

1

The multidimensional nature of pain

LEARNING OUTCOMES

On completion of this chapter, the student will be able to:

■ Critically discuss the physical, psychological and social influences affecting the experience of pain

■ Identify the role of opioid receptors in the management of pain

■ Relate the influence of gating mechanisms to the perception of pain

■ Review the current understanding of tolerance, addiction and dependence

INDICATIVE READING

Bonica, J. (1994) Labour pain. In Wall, P. and Melzack, R. (eds) *Textbook of Pain*, Edinburgh, Churchill Livingstone, pp. 177–91. (For midwifery students.)

Bowsher, D. (1993) Pain management in nursing. In Carrol, D. and Bowsher, D. (eds) *Pain: Management and Nursing Care*, London, Butterworth-Heinemann, Chapter 2.

Clancy, J. and McVicar, A.J. (1995) Pain. In *Physiology and Anatomy: A Homeostatic Approach*, London, Edward Arnold, Chapter 21.

Copp, L.A. (1974) The spectrum of suffering. *American Journal of Nursing*, **74**(3): 491–5.

Dickenson, A. (1995) Novel pharmacological targets in the treatment of pain. *Pain Reviews*, **2**: 1–12.

Fordham, M. and Dunn, V. (1994) *Alongside the Person in Pain: Holistic Care and Nursing Practice*, London, Baillière Tindall, Chapters 1–3.

Hawthorn, J. and Redmond, K. (1998) The physiology of pain and The causes of clinical pain. In *Pain Causes and Management*, Oxford, Blackwell Science, Chapters 2 and 3.

Melzack R. and Wall P.D. (1996) *The Challenge of Pain*, 2nd edn, Toronto, Penguin.

Serpell, M.G., Makin, A. and Harvey, A. (1998) Acute pain physiology and pharmacological targets: the present and future. *Acute Pain*, **1**(3): 31–47.

Sofaer, B. (1998) *Pain: A Handbook for Nurses*, 3rd edn, London, Chapman & Hall.

BACKGROUND

Pain is unlike any other sensation. It is not a single measurable response like blood pressure or pulse; for the person in pain, it is a total experience that cannot be objectively measured. The experience of pain does not depend only on the strength of the stimulus that has caused the painful sensation: an individual's pain perception also depends on how the brain is prepared to deal with the messages it is receiving.

These mechanisms can be subject to huge variation, not only from person to person, but also on a situational basis. They can depend on such factors as:

- a person's mood
- the memory of a previous painful experience
- the cause of the pain and what that might signify to the sufferer
- how one was brought up to view pain
- the time of day and what else is going on around.

All these factors can alter how a painful stimulus is interpreted by the brain. The mechanisms of pain perception are extremely complex, and many attempts have been made to try and explain this phenomenon. This chapter will explore the theoretical basis of pain perception and its relationship to *simple* neurophysiology. We will then consider how this theory relates to people actually experiencing pain. Finally, there are frequent misconceptions regarding the terms 'tolerance', 'addiction' and 'dependency', so it will be important to explore what these terms mean and how they can influence pain management.

WHY HAS PAIN BEEN SO MISUNDERSTOOD?

Ancient philosophers thought of pain as an emotion, an imbalance of body fluids or a visitation from an evil spirit. The heart was seen as the centre of the painful experience. These simplistic theories of pain perception were held until quite recently.

A principle theory was based on the writings of the seventeenth-century philosopher Descartes. He described pain as a spark from a fire that stimulated threads in the skin to operate 'bells' in the brain – a straight channel from the skin to the brain. This simplistic idea of a message travelling directly from the site of pain to the brain has only been challenged in the past 30 years or so, even though the complex layout of nerve pathways was recognised by anatomists a long time ago.

Science has been slow to tackle the problems of pain perception, but science alone is not to blame for this situation: many earlier factors, such as social attitudes to pain and cultural beliefs, have resulted in pain being poorly understood and ineffectively controlled. For centuries, many of these attitudes and beliefs encouraged people to accept that pain was in some way beneficial, character-building or an unavoidable part of disease or injury. Now that we recognise that analgesia and positive pain control strategies – rather than pain – are good for people, we are beginning to see the real benefits of good pain control.

Because pain perception varies widely between and also within individuals, it is possible to understand that Descartes' simple 'hardwired' system cannot possibly be correct; the mechanisms of pain perception are far more complex than this. It was only in 1965 that Professors Melzack and Wall published their paper on a new theory of pain – Gate Control Theory – which was to revolutionise the basic concepts of pain physiology.

Time out   Think about a pain experience you have had.
          What was the cause of the pain?
          Describe the pain – its quality, intensity and location.
          How did it make you feel?

Everyone has at one time or another experienced pain. A recent national survey of hospital patients revealed that 3163 (61 per cent) of patients suffered pain, of whom 1042 (33 per cent) were in pain all or most of the time (Bruster et al., 1994). Pain in the community is difficult to estimate, but some work has been carried out focusing on the pain experienced by patients with cancer. The World Health Organization, for example, conservatively estimated several years ago that at least 4 million people were suffering pain, with or without satisfactory treatment (Foley, 1993). Among the elderly population, the figure can also be alarming, one study revealing that 45–80 per cent of residents in a long-term care facility in the United States suffered from 'significant' pain (Loeb, 1999).

During the previous time out period, were you able to identify what 'type' of pain you have experienced? The first obvious type is either 'acute' or 'chronic'. Acute pain usually has a sudden onset and foreseeable end, and is associated with trauma or acute disease such as appendicitis or cholecystitis. Conversely, chronic pain is usually described as having lasted for more than 3 months, although this is seen by many as being far too simplistic (Waddell, 1997). What is not in dispute is the fact that pain affects many aspects of a person's life – mood, sleep and relationships with other people. Chronic pain might include neuralgic pain and low back pain. Chronic pain may be associated with a degenerative ongoing condition such as osteoarthritis, or, quite frustratingly, it may be associated with no obvious organic pathology at all but still be very real and distressing pain. Other types of pain include tractable/ intractable, persistent/intermittent, referred, somatic, visceral and phantom (see the Glossary at the end of this chapter for definitions of these).

The management of pain will continue to dominate our lives, for several reasons. Painful diseases such as arthritis continue to burden the older age group, in which the numbers are steadily increasing. Also, many people now survive diseases that would once have killed them, and often live with diseases such as cancer. Newer diseases, such as AIDS, emerge and present pain problems for some people.

So how can the theory of pain help us to understand people's pain experience? Gate Control Theory brought together all the current anatomical, physiological, biochemical and psychological data that were available in the 1960s. Despite some modification, the theory has to date stood the test of time and will be covered in greater depth later on. We will initially explore some of the neurophysiology of pain and then consider how Gate Control Theory helps us to understand the lived experience of pain. First of all, it is helpful to define what we actually mean by pain.

Time out   Think about what pain means to you.

Make some notes on how you would describe pain.

Try to write only about what pain is; avoid writing about how it affects you.

Many people have attempted to define pain, and it is helpful to have a definition. McCaffery & Beebe (1994, p. 15) defined pain as:

whatever the experiencing person says it is and existing whenever he says it does.

Another definition is offered to us by the International Association for the Study of Pain (1986):

an unpleasant sensory and emotional experience associated with actual or potential tissue damage, or described in terms of such damage.

What we do know about pain, however, is that it is a subjective experience that is shaped by our previous experiences of pain and is completely individual to the sufferer.

Time out   Think about these two definitions.
How helpful are they to your practice?
Ask a couple of colleagues for their views.

McCaffery's definition is making a statement about always believing the patient. This is fundamental for effective pain management. However, it does little to tell us about the experience of pain, which is clearer in the second definition. The latter also reflects a multidimensional understanding of pain that fits with Gate Control Theory.

AN INTRODUCTION TO NEUROPHYSIOLOGY

Trauma, surgery and inflammatory disease cause a reaction at the site of tissue disruption or damage, and a physiological response throughout the body. The damage to tissue results in the release or production of a mass of chemicals, which react with each other and on nerve endings. This process has been colourfully described as a 'biological nuclear reaction' and the chemicals that result as an 'inflammatory chemical soup'. When these chemicals have stimulated the nerve endings, signals travel to the dorsal horn of the spinal cord and then up to the cortex of the brain, where the perception of pain takes place. For readers who wish to explore this in greater depth, the indicative reading section above provides some sources; for an in-depth text, see Melzack and Wall's (1994) *Textbook of Pain*.

Pain fibres or nociceptors

Looking at the actual nerves themselves, nerves have been classified according to what kind of message they carry, their size and the conduction rates of their fibres. There are three types of nerve fibre that are of particular interest to us. Two carry pain sensation – the A delta and C fibres – the A beta nerves carrying other sensations that are not normally painful, for example warmth and touch.

A delta fibres

When stimulated, these nerves transmit quickly and result in the instant reflex response that will cause the rapid withdrawal of tissue from a source of damage. Imagine putting your hand on the hot plate of a cooker. You remove it so rapidly that you are not consciously aware of your movement. The pain is instant, sharp and localised. This type of sensation carried by the A delta fibres is called 'first' or 'fast' pain.

The fibres travel to the dorsal horn of the spinal cord, which is divided up into layers of cells termed laminae. These laminae have been numbered according to their location. After terminating mainly in lamina 1, the nerves give off long fibres that cross to the other side

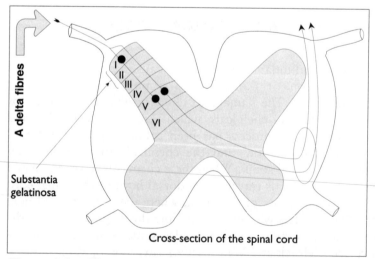

Figure 1.1　The synaptic activity of A delta fibres in the spinal cord

of the cord and then travel to the thalamus and somatosensory areas of the brain cortex (Figure 1.1). Because the A delta fibres end in the 'thinking part' of the cortex, we can fairly accurately localise the pain.

It is these fibres which are also responsible for pinprick sensation. Interestingly, they do not have opioid receptors on their surface. Nurses seem to have known this for a long time as it occurs when a patient who has been made comfortable with morphine is then pricked with a needle. The patient still jumps with the pain: he or she has not been rendered insensible to this sensation just because a previous pain has now been brought under control. This 'first pain' is still intact as a protective mechanism to ensure that tissue is not exposed to further potential damage. It is only by administering a nerve block or rendering a patient deeply anaesthetised that this reflex can be blocked.

Understanding this aspect of pain transmission is important as many patients are left in pain for hours under the mistaken impression that analgesics will 'mask' the pain and make diagnosis more difficult. This is not correct as the tenderness and pain sensation carried by the A delta fibres will not be affected by opioids. When pain has been well controlled but suddenly becomes uncontrolled despite regular, previously effective medication, alarm bells should ring. It could be heralding something serious to cause this change, and the patient's condition should be investigated further.

case history

John Casey is a 28-year-old college student who was admitted to your ward last night with a 24-hour history of nausea and vomiting and right-sided abdominal pain. His general practitioner had given him 10 mg morphine intramuscularly at 3 p.m., and he has received no further analgesia. It is now 9 p.m. and you have just come on night duty. You have found him very distressed and he has rated his pain intensity as 9/10 on a 0–10 scale, 0 being equal to no pain and 10 representing the worst pain ever experienced (see Chapter 2). You notice that his prescription chart has no analgesia prescribed, and the house officer is reluctant to prescribe any until John has been examined by the senior registrar. You are told that John will be going to theatre later this evening. How do you think that you might overcome this problem?

Activity

Talk to colleagues and get them to relate some of their experiences.

Can you make a list of any other situations in which patients might wait in pain unnecessarily? Try making two lists, one covering misconceptions and one covering practice issues (refer to Chapter 5 if you need some help).

An accurate assessment of pain can help with the diagnosis (for example, appendicitis and labour pain), but denying effective analgesia until a diagnosis has been made can result in unnecessary suffering. If an inflamed appendix is painful, morphine will make the patient more comfortable, but if you prod the inflamed area the patient will still complain. It might be helpful to ask for a trial of analgesia for patients like John. This would help medical staff to feel more confident that analgesia, when used appropriately, would not mask the diagnosis yet would offer acceptable pain relief for the patient.

C fibres

These fibres conduct impulses more slowly than A delta fibres and are associated with 'second pain', the dull, burning, aching, throbbing pain that is felt over a wide area usually after the sharp pain. These slower pain fibres terminate in laminae 1 and 2 (the substantia gelatinosa) of the spinal cord and have short connecting fibres to lamina 5 (Figure 1.2).

The C fibres then generally follow the same pathway as the A delta fibres but terminate over a wide area within the brain stem. No fibres project into the somatosensory cortex of the brain, and patients report the pain as being generalised over a wide area. The good news is that this C fibre pain can almost always be subdued by the use of opioid analgesics, which is why this group of pain killer can be so effective in treating acute pain. How opioids achieve this will be covered below.

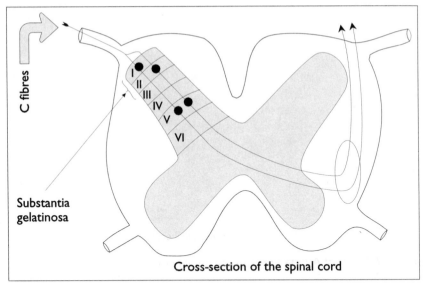

Figure 1.2   The synaptic activity of C fibres in the spinal cord

Non-pain sensation

A beta fibres

Although not directly related to the transmission of painful stimuli, these fibres are worth mentioning here. Like pain fibres, there are many of them, and they are concentrated in the skin. They are the largest of the three fibres, do not cross over to the other side of the spinal cord and are the most rapidly conducting (Figure 1.3). These fibres are activated by touch and sensation that in a normal state would not be perceived as painful. Their significance will become clear when we study Gate Control Theory in more detail.

Figure 1.4 illustrates how the nerve fibres described earlier transmit different sensations. All enter the dorsal horn of the spinal cord at the same point, the A delta and C fibres then crossing over to the other side before travelling up to the brain. The A beta fibres do not cross over but fast-track to the brain on the same side as they enter.

Time out   Think again about pain relief other than that provided by the usual analgesics.

Can you think of specific physical or psychological remedies that work well to relieve pain?

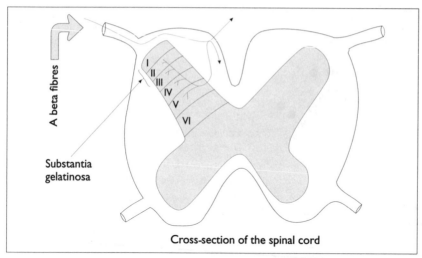

Figure 1.3   Activity of A beta fibres in the spinal cord

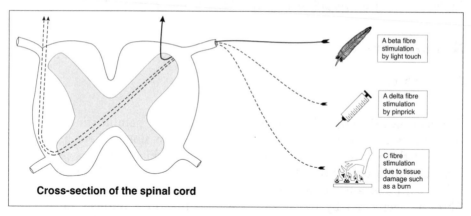

Figure 1.4   Touch, pinprick and burning pain sensations transmitted to the brain via the dorsal horn of the spinal cord

Think about the following everyday scenario. We will then endeavour to explain this process using Gate Control Theory and what is understood about the three nerve fibres that have just been described.

case history

Olivia and Angela are playing at their classmate's fifth birthday party when Olivia falls heavily off the climbing frame. For a moment she is quite shocked and then realises she has hurt her leg. Olivia's mum is nearby and, hearing the cries, scoops her daughter off the ground and cuddles her. When she sees the bruising appearing on Olivia's leg, she gently rubs the affected area, still cuddling her. A few minutes later Olivia is back with her friend, happily playing.

Although there have been several theories to explain the nature of pain, the most influential theory has been Gate Control Theory (Figure 1.5), originally proposed by Melzack and Wall in 1965 and continually updated by further research (Melzack and Wall, 1994). Their theory explains the multidimensional nature of pain, reflecting the physiological, cognitive and emotional aspects of the pain experience, and offers explanations for phenomena that are complex in nature.

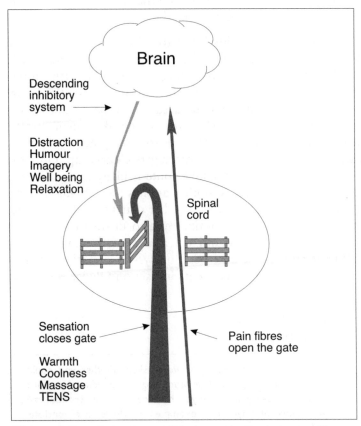

Figure 1.5   Gate Control Theory – how a gate may be opened or closed

Tissue damage results in a volley of nociceptive impulses, which travel along small myelinated A delta nerve fibres and unmyelinated C fibres, these then synapsing with cells in the substantia gelatinosa of the dorsal horn of the spinal cord. If inhibitory impulses do not descend from the brain to close the 'gate', these impulses continue to ascend to the cortex, where the pain is perceived.

A major component of Gate Control Theory is central control, which refers to the influence that cognitive or higher centres of the brain have on pain perception via fibres descending to the 'gating' system. Central activities such as anxiety, excitement and anticipation may open the 'gate' and therefore increase the perception of pain. Conversely, cognitive activities such as distraction, suggestion, relaxation, biofeedback and imagery tend to close the 'gate' and prevent the sensory transmission of pain (Melzack and Wall, 1982). Activation of the faster transmitting A beta fibres, with stimulation such as gentle massage on the affected area, can also close the 'gate' (as happened in the case history when Olivia's mother gently rubbed her leg).

To explain this more easily, think back to Olivia banging her shin, which is hurting. Her mother rubs the developing bruise vigorously but gently. This stimulates the fast-acting A beta fibres (the touch sensation fibres). These then feed into the dorsal horn of the spinal cord, where they synapse in the same area as the pain-transmitting fibres (the substantia gelatinosa). This area is a bit like a major traffic junction: if too many vehicles, in this case too many nerve impulses, arrive at the same time, some of the traffic gets clogged up. Only the swift traffic taking the shortest possible route is likely to get through unhindered. Hence when Olivia's mother applies the rubbing and the warmth that this produces, to the area of her daughter's injured shin, fewer pain sensations reach the brain. By also distracting her with attention and a cuddle, the cognitive features of the gate control mechanism further up the central nervous system are stimulated to help to modulate the pain and reduce its impact on Olivia.

Activity

In a previous Time out, you were asked whether you could think of specific physical or psychological remedies that work well to relieve pain. Now you have covered this section, can you think of any more examples of these interventions reducing the pain experience?

Pain chemicals

Nerve cells have receptors on their surface, which react with or bind to a variety of chemicals found in the 'inflammatory soup' produced by trauma. Some of these chemicals cause the sensation of pain, the principal villains being substance P, bradykinin and the leukotrienes. Once this 'chemical cascade' has commenced, the inflamed tissue and its surrounding area becomes increasingly sensitised to pain by the production of prostaglandins, particularly prostaglandin E. This increase in pain is often termed 'sensitisation'. These chemicals cause the pain transmission to higher centres to increase, thus increasing the pain. Other chemicals can actually reduce pain or remove pain sensation altogether. The action of these chemicals is often referred to as pain 'modulation'. A particularly clear, more in-depth explanation of this complex process can be found in Carr and Goudas (1999).

Activity

Look up the analgesics called non-steroidal anti-inflammatory and make some notes on how they work.

You will find that non-steroidal anti-inflammatory drugs work by inhibiting an enzyme called cyclo-oxygenase, which is responsible for the production of prostaglandin. By inhibiting prostaglandin production, pain intensity is decreased. Unfortunately, one of the downsides of these drugs, usually referred to in abbreviated form as NSAIDs, is their ability to block *all* cyclo-oxygenase enzymes. These include those enzymes needed for the production of the mucosa that protects the stomach and small intestine, as well as chemicals that maintain renal function and platelet adhesiveness (Carr and Goudas, 1999).

One important group of receptors which bind opioid-like chemicals produced in the body are known as the endogenous opioids. Clinicians administer chemicals that mimic these substances in order to reduce pain sensation. These chemicals are able to suppress conduction in the pain pathway and reduce the perception of pain; this is the basis of opioid activity.

13

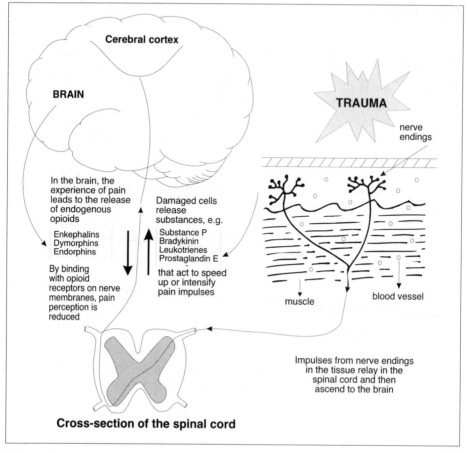

Figure 1.6   Response to the 'chemical cascade' caused by tissue damage

To recap, science has isolated chemicals produced as a result of trauma that can increase pain, but the body also produces opioid-like substances that can alleviate pain. For many thousands of years, man has been aware of a substance that occurs naturally in certain poppies, which can also reduce pain. The opium poppy *Papaver somniferum* produces opium from the sap of its seed head. In the early part of the last century, a young German chemist isolated morphine from the sap of the opium poppy. Morphine is the most powerful analgesic known to man, the 'gold standard' of pain relief and the substance with which other analgesics are compared.

As shown in Figure 1.6, endogenous opioids are morphine-like substances produced by the body. Below is a list of the endogenous opioids that are produced by the body in response to painful stimuli, alongside which are listed some of the commonly administered opioids that are either extracted from opium or manufactured as synthetic copies to produce a similar effect.

Endogenous opioids	Commonly administered opioids	
Enkephalins	Morphine	} extracted from the poppy
Dynorphins	Codeine	
Endorphins	Diamorphine	semi-synthetic compound
	Pethidine	
	Methadone	} synthetic compounds
	Fentanyl	

We will now briefly look at how some of the endogenous opioids and commonly administered opioid drugs actually work.

Opioid receptors

Opioid receptors are principally found in the brain and spinal cord. Opioids (such as those mentioned above) bind to one of three different types of receptor, each receptor having a slightly different action:

1. the *mu receptor* (mu being the 12th letter of the Greek alphabet μ)
2. the *kappa receptor* (after the 10th letter of the Greek alphabet κ)
3. the *delta receptor* (delta being the 4th letter of the Greek alphabet δ).

So far, the majority of the opioid drugs in use are strongly active at the mu receptor. Unfortunately, mu receptor activity produces not only analgesia, but also unwanted side-effects (Table 1.1). A few opioid analgesics act principally on the kappa receptor, producing slightly different, but often no less problematic, side-effects. Table 1.1 shows that delta receptor activity is the only one to produce analgesia alone. This receptor responds to the enkaphalins, but researchers have yet to find a drug that will do the same and result only in analgesia.

Knowing a little more about how opioids work within the body will help you to understand how opioids are most effective in the management of acute pain and can in some cases also be used for specific chronic conditions.

Table 1.1   Activity of opioids at the three receptor sites

Receptor	Response when activated	Endogenous opioid	Analgesic drug with a strong affinity
Mu	Analgesia, respiratory depression, pinpoint pupils, sedation, euphoria, reduced gastric activity, constipation, urinary retention	Endorphins	Morphine
Kappa	Analgesia, dysphoria, hallucinations, paranoia	Dynorphins	Buprenorphine
Delta	Analgesia	Enkephalins	No drug currently available

Figure 1.7 illustrates simply how opioids lock onto the various receptors. When an opioid is firmly locked, it causes an active biological response and is termed an agonist. Although opioids can produce severe unwanted side-effects, administering a substance termed an antagonist can immediately reverse their activity. An antagonist is a substance that can occupy the same receptor but has no biological activity, thus blocking the receptor against the biologically active agonist. For example, if a patient is experiencing respiratory depression as a result of opioid administration and naloxone (an opioid antagonist) is administered, the unwanted side-effect is reversed and the patient's respiratory rate will increase. Unfortunately, if too much naloxone, over and above that needed to restore normal respiratory effort, is given, all analgesic effects are reversed and the pain will inevitably return.

Nurses give out many drugs, for example digoxin, against which there are no antagonists, so why do we get so anxious about the unwanted side-effects of opioids? The fear of respiratory depression and addiction is often given as a reason for health care professionals being reluctant to prescribe and administer opioids. Research, however, indicates these fears are unfounded as fewer than 1 per cent of patients suffer these unwanted side-effects (Friedman, 1990), and every opportunity should be taken to dispel these myths.

For a more in-depth text on opioids, the reader is referred to McQuay (1999).

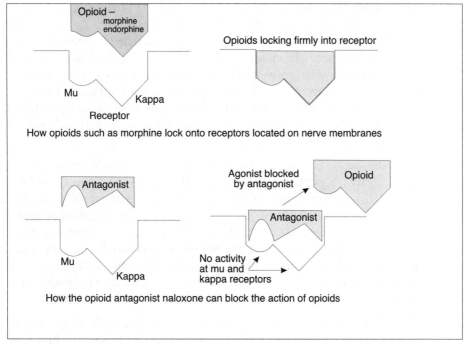

Figure 1.7   Receptor activity

GATE CONTROL THEORY IN UNDERSTANDING THE COMPLEXITY OF PAIN

So far, we have considered several important aspects of neurophysiology that we know contribute to the perception of pain. However, explaining why fast and slow pains are different, as well as the effect that other sensations and chemicals may have on pain perception, does not account for some of the other anomalies that are associated with pain:

- why some people appear to feel pain more than others after the same injury or following the same surgery
- why some people feel pain when there is no apparent injury
- why some people feel no pain when they have a serious injury, for example on a battlefield
- why chronic pain can persist long after the original wound has healed or the initial cause of the pain has been removed
- or even more strangely, why simple touch or stroking can sometimes cause severe pain.

Once again, Melzack and Wall's Gate Control Theory, this time modified, has helped to provide us with an explanation. As mentioned earlier, the dorsal horn of the spinal cord has been subdivided into layers or laminae. Melzack and Wall (1965) recognised that lamina 2 (the substantia gelatinosa) was the site where a major degree of modulation or regulation of the pain pathway took place. This layer receives not only the C fibre and A beta input from the periphery, but also signals from the brain, which travel down the spinal cord and can provide a powerful inhibition of pain.

This discovery is used as the basis for some of our interventions, particularly transcutaneous nerve stimulation (see Chapter 3), and has helped to explain many of the more baffling aspects of pain. The theory also helps to answer the question of why modulation at spinal cord level can have such a profound effect. It is ultimately the brain that dictates how much pain we feel from a potentially noxious stimulus, or whether, in fact, we feel any at all. Wall's book *The Science of Suffering* explains how this works, using a range of fascinating case studies to illustrate how different people do or do not feel pain.

The great strength of Gate Control Theory lies both in the multidimensional framework it offers us and in its plasticity. Plasticity refers to how the peripheral and central nervous systems can be modified and show considerable adaptation to injury (Sluka and Rees, 1997). The sensory-discriminative component of pain allows the injury, as well as its intensity, to be identified in time and space. The affective-motivational (emotional) component relates to how the body reacts to the pain in terms of its protective processes, for example in movement away from the painful stimulus. It is also concerned with how our emotions influence the motivational factors involved in our experience of pain. The final aspect of pain is the cognitive-evaluative component. This explains how our response to painful stimulus is influenced by our cultural values, anxiety, attention and previous pain experience. Gate Control Theory provides a multidimensional explanation for the individual experience of pain, involving all three components. This theory will feature throughout the book so it is important to spend some time understanding it so that you can enjoy using this knowledge as you progress.

Time out   Think back to the pain experience you described at the start of this chapter.

Can you identify any of the components of Gate Control Theory described here?

You might now find it useful to try the following activity. Our personal experience of or preoccupation with some of the points in this activity are believed to influence the descending modulatory mechanism and how the brain responds to a painful stimulus.

Activity

The following active thought processes within the brain influence the descending modulatory mechanism. Try to determine which component of Gate Control Theory (for example cognitive-evaluative) these relate to.

Match the following thought processes to the components of Gate Control Theory by writing in the box opposite.

- Memory of past events

- Boredom

- Emotional state

- Whether the pain is perceived to indicate serious or incurable disease

- Whether attention is being diverted by a more demanding thought process, as is the case on a battlefield or during a crucial rugby match

- How our culture and upbringing may influence our response to pain

- Whether you are being given a massage

ANSWERS

Memory of past events:	predominantly cognitive-evaluative
Boredom:	predominantly cognitive-evaluative
Emotional state:	predominantly affective-motivational
Serious disease:	predominantly affective-motivational
Diverted attention:	predominantly cognitive-evaluative
Culture and upbringing:	predominantly cognitive-evaluative
Massage:	predominantly sensory-discriminatory

Most of the answers will actually involve a combination of the above, again illustrating pain's complexity.

Summary

Not only is pain regulated by the peripheral nervous system (either sensitised by neurotransmitters busily working to increase painful transmission, or modulated by the influence of analgesia, endogenous opioids, touch, vibration and so on), but there is also the possibility of the brain overriding this entire system. This is probably achieved by influencing the release of the transmitters noradrenaline and serotonin within the spinal cord. An increased level of both of these substances would appear to reduce pain. All these factors that sensitise or modulate pain can be thought of as increasing or reducing the volume of pain felt – much as a volume control on a radio regulates sound.

Time out Think about a particular patient whose pain was very difficult to control.

Could the difficulties be explained by the involvement of any or all of the three components of Gate Control Theory?

Pain often becomes difficult to control when a person is very frightened, for example when he or she has lost trust or become overwhelmingly anxious. A combination of other factors may also amplify pain perception, such as feelings of not being in control or not knowing what is happening. A now quite old study by Egbert *et al.* (1964) found that a preoperative discussion of probable postsurgical treatment and possible pain halved the requirement for morphine and reduced the time to discharge. This finding was confirmed in a slightly later study by Hayward (1975) that looked at giving information to patients. Numerous studies have since confirmed these findings.

WHY CAN PAIN GET WORSE WHEN THE DAMAGE APPEARS TO BE HEALING?

The pain a person experiences sometimes seems much worse than would be expected; it may become more intense and widespread than the damage causing it. One of the reasons for this is that prolonged stimulation of the dorsal horn cells within the spinal cord can cause their response to increase, exacerbating the perceived pain. This might happen when someone has experienced a period of intense pain that has not been well controlled. The dorsal horn cells can continue firing long after the stimulus from the periphery has stopped, as when the cause of the pain is no longer evident – when a wound has healed or a broken bone mended, for example. These events are called pain 'wind-up', and in some cases it is thought that prolonged wind-up may result in an acute pain becoming a chronic pain long after the original damage has healed (Gracely *et al.*, 1992).

Tissue damage can also lead to a blurring of the boundaries between the sensations normally carried by A beta fibres and the pain sensations transmitted by C fibres. Pain and sensation fibres both become more easily stimulated, and what would previously have been perceived as an innocuous stimulus to A beta fibres becomes painful. This condition is termed 'secondary hyperalgesia'. The consequences of these changes result in less stimuli proving painful and the pain lasting longer and spreading to uninjured tissue.

Such an outcome is possible because the behaviour of nerves is not fixed. The term 'neural plasticity' is often used when referring to increased pain. It aptly describes the many strange and fascinating activities that can happen within the central nervous system. Evidence is emerging to suggest that wind-up, if allowed to progress, may ultimately be responsible for some acute pain progressing to become a chronic pain syndrome (Dubner and Ruda, 1992).

The possible villain

Although it is not fully understood, it is believed that activation of the NMDA (N-methyl-D-aspartate acid) receptor could be responsible for this unpleasant phenomenon. Many of the chronic pains encountered in pain clinics are thought to be the end-product of this wind-up, pain occurring spontaneously and frequently, and persisting long after healing has taken place (McQuay and Dickenson, 1990).

An understanding of wind-up may help to explain why pre-emptive analgesia, especially when pain is blocked by a local anaesthetic before it enters the spinal cord, often results in such good postoperative analgesia. With the use of opioids, laboratory studies of individual nerve cultures indicate that the activity of these nerves, when treated with low doses of morphine, can be effectively suppressed. As any recovery nurse will tell you, however, once a very painful sensation has reached the conscious brain, it takes a much higher dose of analgesia to suppress the stimulation.

ADDICTION, TOLERANCE AND DEPENDENCE

The literature reveals that health care professionals often hold misconceptions regarding the use of opioids in clinical practice, usually based on a lack of knowledge regarding the mechanisms that come into play when opioids are used regularly. Ferrell *et al.* (1992) reviewed 14 nursing textbooks and discovered that most of them gave inaccurate definitions of addiction, tolerance and dependence.

As there are so many misconceptions regarding the use of opioids, the following section will attempt to clarify some of the issues. For further reading on the subject, refer to the discussion in Melzack and Wall (1994, Ch. 49).

Much of the confusion related to addiction, opioid tolerance and dependence needs to be clarified.

Addiction

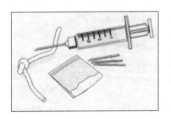 Addiction refers to a psychological dependence characterised by an overwhelming craving for a drug. The addicted individual becomes completely preoccupied with obtaining the drug, but not for its pain-relieving properties. He or she becomes a compulsive drug user who displays loss of control and persistent use despite harm from the drug (Ferrell *et al.*, 1992). The risk of addiction following the use of opioids for pain relief is very small, but many health care professionals are still ignorant of this fact and harbour unnecessary and sometimes irrational fears about addiction.

For example, in a survey of 2459 nurses, over 20 per cent believed that addiction occurred in more than 25 per cent of patients receiving opioids for pain (McCaffery *et al.*, 1990). A further survey in 1992 of 243 US physicians found that 20 per cent believed addiction to be a serious problem in patients with cancer pain (Elliott and Elliott, 1992). However, even when a patient has a prior history of substance abuse, his or her risk of becoming addicted to opioids used for pain relief is very small, probably less than 1 per cent (Ferrell *et al.*, 1992). In a retrospective review of 24,000 patients without a previous history of substance abuse who received opioids for pain relief, approximately 0.3 per cent became addicted. Most of our fears surrounding addiction in patients taking opioids for pain relief are thus completely unfounded. Nevertheless, the mixed messages we all receive as governments and law-enforcement agencies try to curb drug use, often via powerful messages in the media, seems to ensure that many patients will resist the use of opioids for fear of risking addiction.

Tolerance

Patients sometimes appear to get used to a drug and may develop a need for larger doses of opioids in order to control acute, opioid-responsive pain. This does not mean, however, that opioid tolerance is going to become a major problem. In fact, tolerance to some opioid side-effects, such as respiratory depression, occurs normally during long-term administration and enables larger doses of the drug to be administered in order to achieve improved analgesia. Most studies show that, with cancer pain, an increase in analgesia requirement is most probably related to disease progression and increased pain rather than a higher tolerance to the drugs (Collin *et al.*, 1993). Several studies looking at long-term opioid use in patients with advanced cancer show that the longer the duration of treatment, the slower the rate of increase in dose (Twycross and Lack, 1989).

Of nearly 100 advanced cancer patients who received opioids, only 5 per cent of patients required an average daily increase of more than 10 per cent of the previous dose; 81 per cent were said to have a stable dose pattern, and 14 per cent discontinued opioids (Brescia *et al.*, 1992).

Dependence

Physical dependence describes the characteristics of withdrawal symptoms displayed by patients if their opioid dose is significantly reduced or abruptly stopped. These symptoms are not necessarily a feature of long-term opioid use: it is quite possible for patients to display withdrawal symptoms following intensive opioid administration over a relatively short period of time (Melzack and Wall, 1994). Signs of physical withdrawal, which can be very unpleasant for the patient, are easily overcome as long as patients do not discontinue their treatment abruptly. Just as one would with patients who have received another class of drug that mimics substances produced naturally by the body – steroids – it is important to ensure that patients transfer to a tapering dose schedule when opioid dose reduction is indicated.

As previously discussed, the probability of a patient developing addiction and dependence is very remote. It is estimated that addiction occurs in fewer than 0.03 per cent of patients (Porter and Jick, 1980; Ferrell *et al.*, 1992). The best measures to minimise these consequences depend upon an accurate assessment of pain with the patient and then regular monitoring of the efficacy of pain-relieving therapy. This will help health care professionals to select appropriate strategies to manage the pain effectively, ensuring that the dose of drug is appropriate when pain is severe but tapered off once the pain starts to resolve. Working with other health care professionals and helping them to overcome any misconceptions they may have must also be part of the process, in order to ensure effective pain relief.

Activity

Having read the previous section, answer the following questions.

With reference to opioids, what is meant by the terms: 'addiction', 'tolerance' and 'dependence'?

To what extent are these likely to occur during the clinical use of opioids for pain relief, and what measures can be taken to minimise these consequences?

CONCLUSION

This chapter has explored some of the more complex aspects of pain, but hopefully you now have a clearer grasp of the subject that will help you to understand how pain is perceived. Understanding the different mechanisms that contribute to a person's pain experience can help you to select interventions that exploit some of this knowledge and offer more effective pain relief. Fears surrounding addiction often inhibit doctors in prescribing and nurses in administering opioids. Again, understanding the *normal* way in which the body adapts to opioids can dispel these myths and give nurses the confidence to manage pain effectively and educate others.

Pain causes suffering. When an individual is suffering, this will always have an inevitable emotional impact, in turn affecting the sufferer's loved ones and those providing care. Pain always has a psychosocial impact as well as a physiological one. As was once so wisely said, our ability to manage pain effectively is curtailed only by our lack of knowledge (Liebeskind and Melzack, 1987).

After a break, try the multiple-choice questionnaire below in order to self-assess your understanding so far.

Suggested further reading

Cailliet, R. (1994) *Pain: Mechanisms and Management*, Philadelphia, F. A. Davies.

Coniam, S. and Diamond, D. (1994) *Practical Pain Management*, Oxford, Oxford University Press.

Gould, D. and Thomas, V.N. (1997) Pain mechanisms: the neurophysiology and the neuropsychology of pain perception. In Thomas, N.V. (ed.) *Pain: Its Nature and Management*, London, Baillière Tindall, p. 1.

Melzack, R. and Wall, P. (1999) *Textbook of Pain*, 4th edn, Churchill Livingstone. Edinburgh. (An enormous 'pain bible' by the authors of *Gate Control Theory*. Contains every subject on pain for the specialist.)

Park, G. and Fulton, B. (1992) *The Management of Acute Pain*, Oxford, Oxford University Press.(A nice easy to read paperback with a clear description of the pain pathways as we currently understand them.)

The Multidimensional Nature of Pain

MULTIPLE-CHOICE QUESTIONNAIRE

1. Which of the following is thought to modulate pain?

    a. Substance P ☐

    b. Bradykinin ☐

    c. Prostaglandin E ☐

    d. Endorphin ☐

2. Short, sharp pain signals are transmitted by which of the following nerve fibres?

    a. A beta fibres ☐

    b. A delta fibres ☐

    c. C fibres ☐

    d. B delta fibres ☐

3. When opioids reduce pain, which of the following nerve fibres are they affecting?

    a. C fibres ☐

    b. A beta fibres ☐

    c. A delta fibres ☐

    d. B delta fibres ☐

4. The localisation of pain is a function of the:

    a. Substantia gelatinosa ☐

    b. Thalamus ☐

    c. Somatosensory cortex ☐

    d. Dorsal horn ☐

5. Gate Control Theory suggests that pain modulation is the result of:

    a. Stimulation of the spinal cord ☐

    b. Activation of the descending pathways only ☐

    c. Stimulation of the A beta fibres ☐

    d. A combination of A beta fibre stimulation and activation of the descending pathways ☐

6. A cause of pain wind-up is thought to be the activation of which receptor?

    a. GABA ☐   b. NMDA ☐

    c. Kappa ☐   d. Delta ☐

MULTIPLE-CHOICE QUESTIONNAIRE (cont'd)

7. Which of the following statements would reflect a popular definition of opioid addiction?

a. A strong desire to receive an analgesia while experiencing minimal pain ☐

b. An overwhelming psychological drive to take an opioid to experience its psychological rather than pain-relieving effects ☐

c. A compulsion to take an opioid for the fun of it ☐

d. A desire to experience the feeling of euphoria associated with some opioids ☐

8. Which of the following interventions is most appropriate for the management of tolerance in a patient with an opioid-responsive pain?

a. Change the analgesia ☐

b. Keep the dose the same but add another analgesic ☐

c. Stop the analgesics and refer the patient to the clinical psychologist ☐

d. Increase the dose of analgesia until pain control is achieved ☐

9. Which of the following symptoms might suggest physical dependence?

a. When the pain is well controlled, the patient asks for analgesia without any sign of pain ☐

b. Irritability, sweating and anxiety ☐

c. Anxiety and 'clock-watching' ☐

d. The patient requests analgesia regularly ☐

10. How does Gate Control Theory offer us help with selecting interventions?

a. By taking into account the physiological and psychological dimensions of pain, it explains how a variety of interventions may close the gate, thus reducing pain ☐

b. Pain has an affective and cognitive aspect, which means that it will respond to interventions addressing these, for example anxiety reduction and information-giving ☐

c. Pain is just a sensory experience and Gate Control Theory does not help ☐

d. Gate Control Theory suggests that interventions should be psychological ☐

ANSWERS FOR THE MULTIPLE-CHOICE QUESTIONNAIRE

1. **d. Endorphine**; this is the substance produced by the brain that has a pain-relieving action and is sometimes termed an opiate peptide. It is a naturally occurring substance with pharmacological actions resembling morphine.

2. a. **A delta fibres** transmit short, sharp, well-defined pain signals, C fibres generalised dull aching pain and A beta fibres sensations such as vibration and touch. B delta fibres do not exist.

3. a. **C fibres**; there are no opioid receptors located on the A delta fibres that are associated with pain.

4. c. **Somatosensory cortex of the brain**; the substantia gelatinosa is the area in the spinal cord where the modulation of pain occurs. The thalamus is a relay and co-ordinating station for sensory impulses, and the dorsal horn is the area where pain nerve fibres enter the spinal cord before they are relayed to the brain.

5. d. **A combination of A beta fibre stimulation and activation of the descending pathways.**

6. b. **The NMDA receptor**; GABA is thought to be responsible for pain modulation. Kappa and delta are types of opioid receptor.

7. b. **An overwhelming psychological drive to take an opioid to experience its psychological rather than pain-relieving effects.**

8. d. **Increase the dose of analgesia until pain control is achieved**; the other strategies only contribute to causing unrelieved pain and anxiety for the patient.

9. b. **Irritability, sweating and anxiety** are all common symptoms suggesting that the patient has a degree of physical dependence. The sudden cessation of opioids can induce these unpleasant symptoms. Outward signs of pain are notoriously unreliable, and a full pain assessment should always be undertaken before making any assumption. Clock-watching and regular requests for analgesia suggest that pain is poorly controlled and the patient is anxious.

10. a. **By taking into account the physiological and psychological dimensions of pain, it explains how a variety of interventions may close the gate, thus reducing pain.** This explains why interventions that combine pharmacological and non-pharmacological strategies can be so successful. Pain does have an affective and cognitive component (warranting psychological intervention), but it also has a sensory component. Answers c and d are incorrect.

GLOSSARY OF TERMS

Descriptors of pain:

Acute Pain of recent onset and probable limited duration. It usually has an identifiable temporal and causal relationship to injury and disease (IASP, 1986).

Chronic Pain lasting for a long period of time. It usually persists beyond the time of healing of an injury, and there is frequently no identifiable cause (IASP, 1986).

Chronic benign pain Ongoing pain not associated with malignant disease such as cancer.

Chronic malignant pain Pain associated with a life-limiting disease such as cancer.

Intermittent Pain that occurs occasionally or at regular, or irregular, intervals.

Intractable Pain that is difficult to control, influence or alleviate.

Persistent Pain that continues without interruption, being constant and unremitting.

Phantom Pain that is felt to be coming from a limb that has been amputated. The mechanism is not fully understood, but there are suggestions that it might arise from a peripheral origin in the severed nerves in response to changes in the brain or spinal cord.

Referred Pain on the skin is easy to locate, but pain within deep structures is sometimes more difficult of define. Referred pain arises when a visceral organ shares dorsal horn neurones transmitting sensation from the skin; this neurone may then incorrectly interpret the source of the pain.

Somatic Pain in the musculoskeletal system.

Tractable Pain that is easily controlled.

Visceral Pain in the internal organs.

Other:

Affective dimension The emotion associated with thought processes.

Agonist A substance that can act at a cell's receptors. It often mimics the body's normal chemical messenger at this site.

Antagonist A substance that prevents normal activity at a receptor.

Cognitive dimension The thought processes that lead to knowledge, for example perception and reasoning.

Delta The term given to an opioid receptor named after the 4th letter of the Greek alphabet.

Kappa The term given to an opioid receptor named after the 10th letter in the Greek alphabet.

Limbic The system in the brain associated with emotion.

Mu The term given to an opioid receptor named after the 12th letter in the Greek alphabet.

Opioid A generic term for all substances, both natural and synthetic, with a pharmacological action similar to morphine.

2 Assessing Pain

LEARNING OUTCOMES

On completion of this chapter, the student will be able to:

■ Critically evaluate pain assessment tools and measures of pain currently in use for both chronic and acute pain

■ Discuss the importance of implementing pain assessment tools in his or her own clinical area as a means of monitoring individual reports of pain and the efficacy and safety of treatment

■ Review the influence of patient, professional and organisational factors on the effective management of pain

INDICATIVE READING

Baillie, L. (1993) A review of pain assessment tools. *Nursing Standard*, **7**(23): 25–9.

Ho, E. and Heywood, A. (1990) Pain relief in labour. In Alexander, J., Levy, V. and Roth, S. (eds) *Intrapartum Care: A Research-based Approach*, Basingstoke, Macmillan, Chapter 5 (For midwifery students.)

Latham, J. (1994) Assessment and management of pain. *European Journal of Cancer Care*, **3**: 75–8.

McCaffery, M. and Ferrell, B.R. (1997) Nurses' knowledge of pain assessment and management: how much progress have we made? *Journal of Pain and Symptom Management*, **14**(3): 175–88.

Price, D., Bush, F.M., Long, S. and Harkins, S.W. (1994) A comparison of pain measurement characteristics of mechanical visual analogue scale and simple numerical rating scales. *Pain*, **56**: 217–26.

Schofield, P. (1995) Using assessment tools to help patients in pain. *Professional Nurse* **10**(11): 703–6.

BACKGROUND

Evidence suggests that nurses' assessment of pain is limited as well as often being inaccurate (Camp and O'Sullivan, 1987; Zalon, 1993; Carr, 1997a). Nurses still tend to use their own judgement and prefer to rely on physiological signs and behaviours, which can be misleading and inaccurate. Formal pain assessment tools facilitate effective communication and assessment by reducing the chance of error or bias. This chapter explores the nature of pain assessment by critically considering how pain can be assessed and the use of formal pain assessment tools.

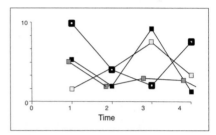

Assessment chart

WHY ASSESS PAIN?

Activity

Take a minute to write down some thoughts on this question.

If you are to manage pain effectively, it is imperative that you use a pain assessment tool rather than ask vague questions from the drug trolley, such as 'Anything for pain, Mr Jones?' A district nurse may elicit very little information if asking closed questions such as 'Have you any pain? This does not constitute a pain assessment and may even inhibit a truthful answer as patients may feel that they cannot talk about their pain. However, adequate assessment without effective management strategies will result in poor-quality care. Some of the advantages of using a formal pain assessment tool are that it:

● provides patients with an opportunity to express their pain
● conveys genuine concern and interest about their pain
● helps to build a therapeutic relationship
● gives patients an active role in their pain management
● provides documented evidence of the efficacy or failure of any drugs or therapy provided
● enables the incidence of any side-effects to be documented and their treatment evaluated

- reduces the chances of bias and error
- helps communication with other health professionals.

Can you think of any other advantages of incorporating pain assessment into the general monitoring of patients?

Activity

Approach a person you know is experiencing pain or discomfort.

Ask them if they are happy to discuss their pain.

Find out what increases or reduces their pain.

Make some notes about what they say; we will revisit these notes at the end of this section.

It is not possible to measure pain objectively in the clinical setting as we would measure a blood pressure; instead, we must mainly rely on subjective verbal methods. When communication with the patient is difficult, the observation of non-verbal communication and physiological responses is the only alternative. Assessment tools to help to assess these non-verbal indicators of pain are being developed, and many are currently in use to assess pain in infants and small children. These tools are covered in greater depth in Chapter 6, but there is still a long way to go in their development so there is plenty of scope for creativity.

WHEN TO ASSESS PAIN

Pain assessment should ideally be integrated into the admission procedure or initial health assessment, which can be especially useful for patients prior to surgery, for example. They might have pain that was not previously documented, the nurse can obtain some information about how they have managed pain in the past, previous experiences may be relevant and knowing their expectations of pain management can be useful. A proactive approach has several advantages:

- On admission, discussing pain assessment offers the opportunity to provide information to those patients who may find this beneficial (Shade, 1992).
- Patient misconceptions can constitute a serious barrier to good pain management (Carr, 1997a). It is useful to be aware of these misconceptions before commencing any therapy. Unfounded fears of addiction can seriously hamper even the best efforts to control pain.
- The nurse will be able to identify important issues that will improve pain assessment and management.
- Previous pain experiences can influence patients' expectations of how their pain will be managed.
- The suitability of a pain assessment tool can be checked before it is used. This is particularly important with children who might prefer to use a 'faces' scale rather than a verbal or numerical scale.
- For non-verbal patients, a discussion with family or carers may help when selecting or modifying a pain assessment tool.
- Now is a good time to stress to the patient that pain is not considered to be an inevitable part of being a patient and that there are plenty of ways to control pain.

HOW TO ASSESS PAIN

Verbal communication

Where possible, verbal assessment is the best form of assessment; this is the principal method unless a patient's age or condition makes it impossible. Assessment should commence as early as possible, for example preoperatively, as it can be valuable to establish the patient's expectation of pain relief. This is unfortunately often very low. People frequently come into hospital expecting pain from operations, tests or investigative procedures. Sadly, we usually give them what they expect, so on satisfaction surveys, patients are satisfied with their care. Even when patients have memories of considerable pain, they still report being satisfied with their pain relief as they got what they expected... *pain*.

Communication is vital if the situation is going to improve, and it must be a two-way process. The patient must be provided with suitable information regarding the various pain-relieving therapies that are available, and information must be obtained on patients' expectations of pain relief. It is also important to inform patients of the benefits of effective pain control, for example to allow them to mobilise or cough, and to prevent unwanted side-effects. Too often, patients will resist taking analgesia and think that as long as they keep still and do not move, they will not experience pain. Unfortunately, it is this immobility which can lead to sometimes life-threatening side-effects such as deep vein thrombosis and chest infection.

Visual displays of pain

With patients unable to communicate verbally, for whatever reason, the nurse will have to rely on visual and physical signs of pain. As unlikely as it may seem, even fully verbal patients may not wish verbally to communicate that they are in pain. They might, for example, fear that a report of pain could lead to them spending more time in hospital, or they might be denying their pain for fear of what that pain might signify. In such cases, non-verbal displays of pain may be useful. For the neonate or non-verbal, cognitively impaired patient, visual displays of pain may be all that is available in order to assess pain. (Chapter 6 covers the management of these vulnerable patients in more detail.) Visual signs might include:

- *body language:* limited movement or keeping very still, guarding parts of the body, an abnormal posture, a change in gait when walking or a change in stature, rocking, picking and restlessness
- *facial expression:* increased or decreased eye contact, tears, grimacing, muscle tension, an alarmed look, squinting eyes and clenched teeth
- *vocalisation:* sighing, crying, moaning, spontaneous noises, a change in pitch, impaired speech, verbal abuse, disjointed verbalisation and calling out
- *distance:* becoming quiet, withdrawn and uncommunicative
- *emotion:* worried looking, angry, sad or a change in mood
- *other:* a lack of interest in food and the environment, or a disrupted sleep pattern.

Physical signs of pain

Changes in physiological signs can support the patient's report of pain but should not (except in the unconscious patient) be used as the only measure as patients eventually adapt to pain.

- *physiological:* relative changes in blood pressure (up or down), pulse and respiration rate, sweating, pallor and nausea
- *physical:* in chronic pain, changes in limb size as a result of muscle wasting, neurological abnormalities, changes in temperature and colour, mottling of the skin of an affected limb or muscle spasm.

case history

Clive is an elderly gentleman who has been admitted to your ward with widespread cancer metastases. He is quiet, withdrawn and unable to concentrate for long. Clive frequently grimaces and moans. Because of the onset of severe nausea in the past 48 hours, he has been unable to take his regular oral analgesia – 100 mg slow-release morphine every 12 hours with 6-hourly paracetamol. What information do you need in order to plan your care effectively?

Possible solution: You will need to assess the pain quickly and with the least number of questions. Tell the patient that, in order to obtain effective analgesia, you will need to ask a few questions but that you will keep them brief.

1. Get the patient to indicate the location of the pain.

2. Ask how long the pain has been there.

3. Ask the patient to rate the severity of his pain on a scale of 0–10 (0 = no pain and 10 = worst pain imaginable). Remember that not everyone will be able to give a numerical rating: they may be unable to concentrate, or they may not understand the concept. A simple verbal rating, although less sensitive, is then more appropriate, taking, for example, the form 'Is your pain now mild, moderate or severe?'

4. Ask the patient what he normally takes for his pain and any strategies he finds helpful.

With this minimal information, you will have established the location, duration and severity of the pain, as well as the dose of medication that would normally provide relief. While his nausea is being brought under control, his opioid intake can be re-established via a non-oral route, that is, intravenously, subcutaneously, rectally or sublingually.

NURSE FACTORS AFFECTING THE ASSESSMENT OF PAIN

There is a need for nurses to be aware of how their own values and perceptions may influence the evaluation of another person's response to pain. If health care professionals hold misconceptions or anxieties regarding pain management, these must be addressed through education. McCaffery (1991) discovered that nurses were, when making a pain assessment, strongly influenced by patients' behaviour. This was confirmed by Allcock (1996), who conducted a literature review on the factors affecting the assessment of postoperative pain. To explore this subject further, see Carr (1997a).

PATIENT FACTORS AFFECTING THE ASSESSMENT OF PAIN

A person's age, gender, previous experience of pain and cultural background all influence pain perception. Nurses need to be aware of these influences and remain non-judgemental and unbiased in their assessment of another person's pain. It is important to be aware that pain behaviours may not always indicate the 'level' of pain that a person is feeling. People experiencing pain may try to minimise their pain; they may not want to worry their family, they may be embarrassed, they may feel that it is better to bear the pain or worry that it may stop them going home from hospital, or they may harbour other misconceptions about pain and its management. Briggs (1995) presents an interesting paper that has explored the literature on patient factors influencing the expression of pain and highlights these in relation to acute pain assessment. Some of these are now explored.

Age

The elderly

Elderly people may 'hide' their pain, especially if it is chronic. At home, they may have developed good strategies to help them through the day. Sadly, when they are admitted to hospital, these disappear and patients are left vulnerable and often unable to cope with their pain. The 'obvious' pain behaviours such as grimacing and frowning are often absent if pain has been chronic. In addition, sufferers may feel that it is not 'acceptable' to express their pain or that it is a sign of weakness. Nurses need a knowledge of the expression of pain in this population if they are to recognise and manage it successfully. An informative and thought-provoking article by Hayes (1995) considers the lack of research and the difficulties in assessing pain in elderly people, especially when there is confusion or the person is unable to respond verbally.

case history

Joan is suffering from dementia and has been admitted to a rehabilitation ward for respite care while her daughter takes a few days' holiday. Joan initially settled well, but after a few days you notice that she is reluctant to sit in her chair and is constantly fidgeting and trying to get comfortable. When you ask her whether she has any pain, she nods but is unable to respond verbally. You noticed earlier that it took a couple of nurses to help her out of bed this morning, and her right hip seemed particularly stiff. Make notes on how you might assess Joan's pain.

Possible solution:

1. In an ideal situation, a preassessment with Joan's daughter might have enabled you to list any behaviour that she felt might indicate pain.

2. Make a brief list of the behaviours you observe when Joan is being moved or appears to be uncomfortable.

3. Observe her facial expression and body movements.

4. The fact that Joan nods in response to your question about pain means that it may be quite possible for you to obtain a regular self-report of pain using a simple pain assessment tool. If everything is explained carefully, it is often quite surprising how effectively patients, even those with severe cognitive impairment, can communicate pain, if they are given the chance.

5. Try to identify any new pathology, worsening of known pathology or procedures that appear to cause pain.

6. Give a trial of analgesia and observe Joan's response. Does she appear more comfortable and relaxed, or is she still displaying discomfort, which could also be related to her sudden change of scenery and the anxiety that this might be causing.

7. Read Chapter 7 of this book for some more information on pain assessment tools for the cognitively impaired.

Small children and neonates

Very small children seem historically to have had their pain even more poorly managed than have adults. Nagy (1998) studied the effect that this had on the psychological state of nurses looking after neonates. The study revealed that a primary source of stress among these nurses was the lack of valid assessment tools. We are now, thankfully, beginning to make some progress in this field.

Gender

Another factor that has been extensively discussed is gender and its impact on pain experience. Despite several studies, however, the results are inconclusive (Feine *et al.*, 1991; Bush *et al.*, 1993).

Activity

Ask a few friends or patients who they think feel pain more (men or women).

Make a note of their responses.

How could this influence the management of pain in practice?

See whether you can find any literature on the subject. The use of vignettes in research would seem to indicate that many of us hold preconceived ideas.

Women who have given birth, and experienced intense pain, may be better able to cope with pain when they next experience it, especially if they felt in control at the time. It might also be argued that it is more acceptable for women than men to express their pain in an Anglo-Saxon-based culture. This might mean in practice that women 'appear' to suffer more pain than men if we are judging a person's pain by their behaviour.

PAIN ASSESSMENT SCALES

To capture formally from patients information on their pain, a pain assessment tool is used. The pain assessment tool should ideally be valid, that is, there should be evidence that the tool is useful for the purpose intended, reliable and easily understood by the patient. For acute pain, which may change frequently, the assessment tool also needs to be fairly quick to use. The following section considers a range of different types of tool, including rating scales, the London Hospital Pain Chart and the Short-form McGill Pain Questionnaire. Pain assessment should also include the family or immediate carer. They will have a valuable insight into and understanding of the patient's pain experience, especially if there is cognitive impairment, hearing or visual difficulty.

The most reliable indicator of a person's pain and the distress it may be causing them is the patient's self-report. Self-report measurement scales include numerical or descriptive rating scales and visual analogue scales. A pain intensity score is a quick way of finding out the intensity of the pain for a given individual and evaluating the effectiveness of an intervention. Such scores are usually quick and simple to use, and most patients are able to understand them. The disadvantage of these scales is that they measure only intensity and give neither a description of the pain nor any additional information.

Visual analogue scale

This scale incorporates a 10 cm line, one end labelled 'No pain at all' and the other end labelled 'Worst pain imaginable' (Figure 2.1). Patients are asked to mark on the line the point corresponding to their pain. A pain score is then obtained by measuring, usually in millimetres, the distance between 'No pain at all' and the patient's mark. This can then give a precise figure and, when repeated later, can indicate small changes in pain intensity. This scale requires a patient to be able to concentrate. Some may have trouble understanding the concept, especially immediately postoperatively, or if they are cognitively impaired.

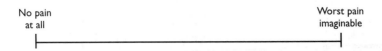

Figure 2.1   Visual analogue scale

Simple descriptive and numerical scales

These were the earliest of the pain assessment tools and quite simply use words, numbers or a combination of words and numbers to indicate the intensity of the pain or the effectiveness of any pain-relieving measures (Figure 2.2). They are easy to explain to patients and can be asked as a simple question.

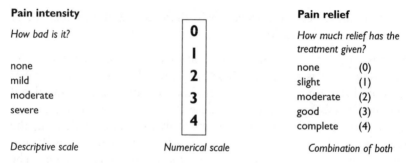

Pain intensity

How bad is it?

none
mild
moderate
severe

Descriptive scale

0
1
2
3
4

Numerical scale

Pain relief

How much relief has the treatment given?

none   (0)
slight   (1)
moderate   (2)
good   (3)
complete   (4)

Combination of both

Figure 2.2   Examples of pain scales

London Hospital Pain Chart

The London Hospital Pain Chart (Figure 2.3; Raiman, 1986) was developed with the aim of improving communication between the patient, the nurse and the doctor. The chart incorporates a body map, which has been shown to be particularly useful in pinpointing the source of pain (Latham, 1989). There are clear instructions on how to complete the chart, and simple pain interventions are included. It is

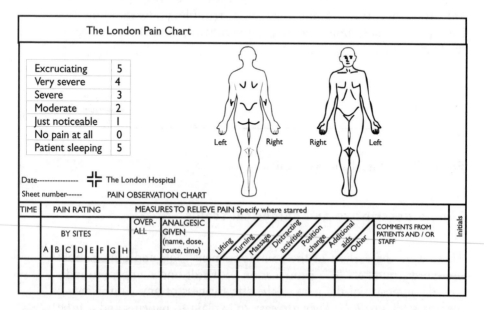

Figure 2.3   London Hospital Pain Chart (Reproduced by kind permission of Mark Allen Publishing)

helpful if patients can indicate their pain on the body map as it encourages them to participate actively in the pain assessment process.

Short-form McGill Pain Questionnaire

Melzack and Torgerson (1971) suggested that the words people chose to express their pain could form the basis of a pain assessment tool. The McGill Pain Questionnaire (MPQ) is now one of the most utilised pain assessment tools in both research and clinical practice, and is particularly helpful across a range of painful conditions, particularly chronic pain. Figure 2.4 displays the short-form version (SF-MPQ).

The MPQ comprises a list of 78 words categorised into 20 groups that represent four major dimensions of pain quality: sensory, affective, evaluative and miscellaneous. Each word has a score value, and the patient is asked to select words that describe his or her pain. The short-form of the MPQ, illustrated in Figure 2.4 takes less than 5 minutes to complete and is sensitive to clinical change resulting from pain interventions, for example analgesia (Melzack, 1987).

Several scores can be calculated using the MPQ. For example, the total value of the words chosen gives the Pain Rating Index (PRI) for each of the dimensions – sensory, affective, evaluative and miscellaneous. These can also be added together to give the PRI-Total. The total number of words chosen (NWC) is another score, and there is also the Present Pain Intensity (PPI), which is an intensity score derived from a 0–5 scale. This is a useful tool for gaining a broader perspective of the patients' experience of pain and how it is affecting them. Although primarily used in chronic pain, it has been successfully used with acute pain sufferers. For further information regarding these pain assessment tools, see Melzack and Katz (1994).

Pain Diaries

Asking patients to keep a diary of their pain can be very helpful to gain an understanding of factors which might exacerbate or reduce their pain. In the community they might be particularly useful and patients often enjoy the activity and feel they are participating in their care more fully.

Patient's name . . . .   Date . . . .

	None	Mild	Moderate	Severe
Throbbing	0)	1)	2)	3) . . . . . .
Shooting	0)	1)	2)	3) . . . . . .
Stabbing	0)	1)	2)	3) . . . . . .
Sharp	0)	1)	2)	3) . . . . . .
Cramping	0)	1)	2)	3) . . . . . .
Gnawing	0)	1)	2)	3) . . . . . .
Hot-burning	0)	1)	2)	3) . . . . . .
Aching	0)	1)	2)	3) . . . . . .
Heavy	0)	1)	2)	3) . . . . . .
Tender	0)	1)	2)	3) . . . . . .
Splitting	0)	1)	2)	3) . . . . . .
Tiring/exhausting	0)	1)	2)	3) . . . . . .
Sickening	0)	1)	2)	3) . . . . . .
Fearful	0)	1)	2)	3) . . . . . .
Punishing/cruel	0)	1)	2)	3) . . . . . .

No pain ⟵———————————————⟶ Worst possible pain

PPI

0 No pain   . . . .

1 Mild   . . . .

2 Discomforting   . . . .

3 Distressing   . . . .

4 Horrible   . . . .

5 Excruciating   . . . .

Descriptors 1–11 represent the sensory dimension of the pain experience and 12–15 the affective dimension. Each descriptor is ranked on an intensity scale of 0 = none, 1 = mild, 2 = moderate and 3 = severe. The present pain intensity (PPI) of the standard Long-form McGill Pain Questionnaire (LF-MPQ) and the visual analogue scale are also included to provide an overall intensity score.

Figure 2.4   Short-form McGill Pain Questionnaire (SF-MPQ) (Reproduced by kind permission of R. Melzack)

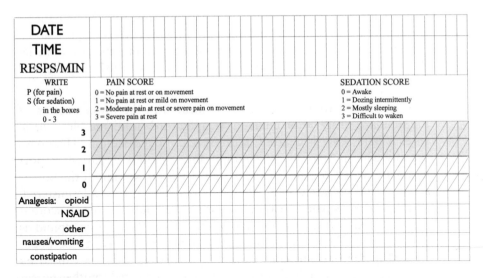

Figure 2.5   Chart for recording acute pain intensity

Time out   Pain is frequently inadequately assessed. We know that failure to assess pain is a major barrier to its effective control, but few hospitals include pain assessment in their routine patient monitoring. What strategies might encourage practitioners to assess pain? Discuss this with colleagues and see whether you can come up with any suggestions.

Charts used for regular everyday use

Getting practice to change is not an easy feat. Pain management and its inadequacies have long been reported, and it has been suggested that one of the reasons why practice has been slow to change is the lack of institutionalised policies that could positively affect pain management.

Figure 2.5 comprises a chart introduced into a district general hospital some years ago to enable the routine assessment of acute pain to be documented on standard monitoring charts on the wards. Although it is fairly straightforward, its use is still sporadic and unsatisfactory. It would seem that nurses still assume that patients will tell them when they are in pain, although this rarely happens in reality. Most patients expect the nurse to know that they are in pain and to enquire about their pain, so we are left with a fundamental communication barrier that can prove very difficult to remove (Seers, 1987; Franke and Theeuwen, 1994).

The assessment tool in Figure 2.5 is located in the lower portion of the standard observation chart for temperature, pulse and blood pressure. A pain score is charted in the special boxed section. The boxes are divided in two by a diagonal line. Should a patient report moderate or severe pain, this is scored in the top section of the box as a 2 or 3 and indicated by the letter P. Analgesia is then administered, and the patient's pain is reassessed within the hour. The repeat score is then charted in the bottom half of the box. If a strong opioid is administered, the chart enables the sedation score also to be documented in the bottom half of the box. Excessive sedation caused by too large a dose of opioid is then easily communicated to other nurses as the monitoring chart and drug chart are clipped together at the end of the patient's bed. The chart forms part of a periodic audit against a hospital standard that no patient experiences moderate or severe acute pain for more than 1 hour.

The development of this chart was part of a hospital-wide policy to raise the profile of pain management and incorporate an 'institutionalised' practice to encourage nurses regularly to monitor and document pain assessment. It was hoped that by having pain assessment on a standard observation chart, pain would be assessed regularly.

CHANGING PRACTICE – INTRODUCING A PAIN ASSESSMENT TOOL

Selecting a pain assessment tool for use in clinical practice requires careful consideration. The article by Baillie (1993) reviews a few more tools; see whether any seem particularly useful for your clinical area and then complete the activity opposite.

You have probably found out from your various activities that, for acute pain, you need a simple tool to assess the site of the pain and its intensity. For chronic pain, however, considerably more information is needed. It is unusual to assess chronic pain on a regular basis such as 4-hourly so far more information is usually incorporated into the chart. Not only are site and intensity important, but other factors could also be particularly significant. We need to know what the pain feels like and

Activity

Choose one pain assessment tool that you feel would be appropriate for your client group.

Assess the pain of between 5 and 10 clients (you might want to modify the tool a little).

When assessing their pain, consider how 'good' the tool is at accurately identifying the level and type of the pain. Make notes about how easy the tool was to use, how long it took to administer and what the client felt about you using the tool. Did you get any surprises?

Think about the patient you interviewed at the start of this unit.

How did the information differ when you were assessing pain with a formal tool compared to when you asked casual questions?

how often it occurs. Is it there constantly; what are the aggravating or relieving factors? How does the pain affect the way in which a patient feels, and what impact does the pain have on a patient's quality of life? What is the duration of the pain? Finally, a tool that enables the documentation of all the strategies that are helpful, both pharmacological and non-pharmacological, will lead to good communication and ensure that previously unhelpful strategies are not reintroduced.

Activity

For some people who live with chronic pain day in, day out, assessing their pain might be detrimental.

Why is this, and what could you do to ensure that assessment did not result in a worsening of their ability to cope with their pain?

People experiencing chronic pain often use successful strategies such as distraction to minimise their pain; regular questions about their pain may, however, reduce the effectiveness of this distraction. With chronic pain, especially when a cure is unlikely, assessment may take place on a daily, weekly or even less frequent basis. New treatments or therapies will need fairly frequent evaluation, but regularly making a patient refocus on his or her chronic pain could be counterproductive.

CONCLUSION

Pain assessment and documentation is essential to the effective management of pain. This chapter has explored the process of pain assessment and considered not only factors that can affect an individual's perception and expression of pain, but also pain assessment tools that can be utilised in clinical practice. Convincing practitioners of the importance of pain assessment tools can be a difficult process, yet it is of paramount importance that pain assessment is incorporated into daily practice, whether it be in hospital or in a community setting. Bias, stereotyping and the inaccurate collection of information can all contribute to errors in assessment (Harrison, 1991). An accurate, sensitive and detailed assessment forms the foundation of effective management.

After a break, try the multiple-choice questionnaire below in order to self-assess your understanding so far.

Suggested further reading

Albrecht, M.N., Cook, J.E., Riley, M.J. and Andreoni, V. (1992) Factors influencing nurses' decisions for non-documentation of patient reponse to analgesia. *Journal of Clinical Nursing*, 1: 243–51.

Camp, D. (1987) Comparison of medical, surgical and oncology patients' descriptions of pain and nurses' documentation of pain assessments. *Journal of Advanced Nursing*, 12: 593–8.

Carrol, D. and Bowsher, D. (1993) *Pain Management and Nursing Care.* Butterworth-Heinemann. (See Chapter 3.)

Fordham, M. and Dunn, V. (1994) *Alongside the Person in Pain*, London, Baillière Tindall. (See Chapter 4.)

Harrison, A. (1991) Assessing the patients' pain: identifying reasons for error. *Journal of Advanced Nursing*, **16**: 1018–25.

Hunt, K. (1995) Perceptions of patients' pain: a study assessing nurses' attitudes. *Nursing Standard*, **5**(2): 14–16.

McCaffery, M. and Beebe, A. (1994) *Pain: Clinical Manual for Nursing Practice*, London, C.V. Mosby. (See Chapter 2.)

Pearce, C. (1993) Formal measurement of pain by nurses. *Nursing Standard*, **7**(21): 38–9.

Raiman, J. (1986) Monitoring pain at home. *Journal of District Nursing*, **4**(11): 4–6.

Walker, J. (1992) Taking pains (attitudes for pain assessment) *Nursing Times*, **88**(29): 38–40.

Walker, J. (1994) Caring for elderly people with persistent pain in the community: a qualitative perspective on the attitudes of patients and nurses. *Health and Social Care*, **2**: 221–8.

Watt-Watson, J. and Donovan, M. (1992) *Pain Management: Nursing Perspective*, St Louis, C.V. Mosby Year Book. (See Chapter 4.)

Pain Assessment

MULTIPLE-CHOICE QUESTIONNAIRE

1. What factors contribute to the inaccurate assessment of pain?

    a. Nurses do not use pain assessment tools ☐

    b. Nurses rely on their own judgement and on patient behaviours ☐

    c. Patients are unwilling to discuss their pain ☐

    d. Doctors do not use pain assessment tools ☐

2. Many common misconceptions are held about pain. Which of the following statements is correct?

    a. Patients in pain always have observable signs ☐

    b. Patients will always tell a nurse when they have pain ☐

    c. Patients are the experts on their pain ☐

    d. Pain is part of being unwell ☐

3. Elderly patients often hide their pain. Which of the following reasons is incorrect?

    a. They have often developed good coping strategies ☐

    b. Over time, the obvious pain behaviour disappears ☐

    c. They may feel that expressing their pain will be seen as a sign of weakness ☐

    d. Pain intensity decreases with age, and therefore their pain is not as severe ☐

MULTIPLE-CHOICE QUESTIONNAIRE (cont'd)

4. Several factors are known to affect pain assessment. Which of the following factors is not implicated?

  a. The patient's age, gender and previous experience of pain ☐

  b. The nurse's previous experience of pain ☐

  c. The patient's ability to communicate ☐

  d. Health professionals rather than the patient are knowledgeable about pain ☐

5. Pain assessment tools must fulfil a number of criteria. Which of the following is most desirable?

  a. They must be valid, reliable and easily understood by the patient ☐

  b. They must be reliable and quick to use ☐

  c. They should measure only the intensity of the pain ☐

  d. They should measure both chronic and acute pain ☐

6. Which pain assessment tool is the most effective for the measurement of pain intensity?

  a. A verbal rating scale ☐

  b. A visual analogue scale ☐

  c. A 'faces' rating scale ☐

  d. A physiological assessment ☐

7. How many scores can be calculated for the McGill Pain Questionnaire?

  a. Two ☐   c. Seven ☐

  b. Four ☐   d. Three ☐

8. Which activity could positively influence effective pain assessment?

  a. Asking patients to complete their own assessment charts ☐

  b. Institutionalising pain assessment – making it a hospital policy regularly to assess and document pain ☐

  c. Regular visits by pain teams ☐

  d. More time ☐

9. If someone is experiencing chronic pain, why might regular assessment be detrimental?

  a. It is too time-consuming ☐

  b. By focusing on the pain, it reduces patients' coping strategies ☐

  c. It encourages patients to exaggerate their pain ☐

  d. There is little that can be done to manage chronic pain ☐

MULTIPLE-CHOICE QUESTIONNAIRE (cont'd)

10. To complement the data collected by a verbal rating pain assessment tool, what other information might you need?

a. Blood pressure, pulse rate and respiratory rate ☐

b. A medical and family history ☐

c. Any previous experience of pain, and the coping strategies used ☐

d. Observation of the patient's behaviour ☐

ANSWERS FOR THE MULTIPLE-CHOICE QUESTIONNAIRE

1. b. **Nurses rely on their own judgement and on patient behaviour**; evidence suggests that nurses do not use formal assessment tools that would help patients to communicate a subjective experience. Instead, they rely on their own judgement and patients' behaviour. If a patient is not demonstrating overt 'pain behaviour' (for example, grimacing or becoming withdrawn), nurses may wrongly assume that they are not experiencing pain.

2. c. **Patients are the experts on their pain**; patients should not expect to have pain while in hospital, although unfortunately many do. Observable signs of pain are extremely unreliable, and a large number of patients will not report when they are in pain: they will expect the nurse to know about their pain.

3. d. **Pain intensity decreases with age, and therefore their pain is not as severe**; research has shown that this is not true, although many clinicians still believe this to be the case. In the older adult, many factors may inhibit people expressing their pain, especially if it is chronic. They may, for example, feel that it is not acceptable to express pain, or that it is something they have to bear. This may be coupled with difficulties in communication, which only compound the problem.

4. d. **Health care professionals rather than the patient are knowledgeable about the pain** is a belief which hampers accurate pain assessment. All the other factors mentioned can affect the quality and accuracy of a pain assessment. The nurse's own experience of pain can influence how she assesses pain and should be recognised in order to avoid a biased assessment.

5. a. **They must be valid, reliable and easily understood by the patient**; these are the most desirable features of a good pain assessment tool. Some pain assessment tools, such as the MPQ, will take longer to complete, but the nature of the pain may necessitate this. Pain is multidimensional, and a pain assessment tool should reflect this. Some tools, for example visual analogue scales, may be better for acute pain while others, for example the MPQ, may be more suited to chronic pain.

6. b. **A visual analogue scale** will provide the sensitivity when it comes to measuring pain intensity. Verbal ratings are good for determining the quality of the pain.

49

Physiological assessment tools only assist an educated guess, and the 'faces' rating scale includes only six progressive levels, which limits the choices available.

7. c. **Seven,** comprising the total value of the words from the four dimensions (sensory, affective, evaluative and miscellaneous) which can be added together to give the PRI-Total, the total number of words chosen and the PPI.

8. b. **Institutionalising pain assessment – making it a hospital policy regularly to assess and document pain**; attempts to improve pain assessment and management have often failed because they have not become part of hospital policy and procedure. Incorporating a pain assessment tool into observation charts would encourage regular assessment and documentation. Although an increased number of visits from the pain team might be beneficial, it might also reduce the ward nurses' perceived responsibility for pain management.

9. b. **By focusing on the pain, it reduces patients' coping strategies**; when someone is using distraction to take their mind off pain, regular assessments can break this coping strategy and cause them to focus on their pain again. Regular pain assessment need not be time-consuming, especially if patients are encouraged to participate in the process. It is unlikely that they will exaggerate their pain: they are in fact more likely to minimise it. There are many interventions for chronic pain that have been shown to help people to cope with their pain.

10. c. **Any previous experience of pain, and the coping strategies used**; ascertaining these is invaluable in gaining a better understanding of the meaning of pain for this person and how best to incorporate previous interventions that have been helpful. Physiological and behavioural observations are notoriously unreliable. The medical and family history may or may not be directly related to the current pain experience. In addition, people may experience pain when there is no evident pathology.

3 Managing acute pain

LEARNING OUTCOMES

On completion of this chapter the student will be able to:

■ Review the psychological, behavioural and physical strategies used in the management of acute pain

■ Critically evaluate current methods of pain management and their use in institutional and non-institutional settings

■ Analyse practices for managing acute pain in his or her own clinical area and identify methods of influencing change

INDICATIVE READING

Carr, D.B. and Goudas, L.C. (1999) Acute pain, *Lancet*, **353**: 2051–8.

Kitson, A. (1994) Postoperative pain management: a literature review. *Journal of Advanced Nursing*, **3**: 7–18.

Mather, C. and Ready, B. (1994) Management of acute pain. *British Journal of Hospital Medicine*, **51**(3): 85–8.

Moore, S. (ed.) (1997) *Understanding Pain and its Relief in Labour*, Edinburgh, Churchill Livingstone. (For midwifery students.)

Pediani, R.C. (1998) Organising acute pain management. In Carter, B. (ed.) *Perspectives on Pain, Mapping the Territory*, London, Arnold, Chapter 12.

Royal College of Surgeons of England and College of Anaesthetists (1990) *Report of the Working Party on Pain after Surgery*, London, HMSO.

Scott, N.B. and Hodson, M. (1997) Public perceptions of postoperative pain and its relief. *Anaesthesia*, **52**: 438–42.

Seers, K. and Carroll, D. (1998) Relaxation techniques for acute pain management: a systematic review. *Journal of Advanced Nursing*, **27**(3): 466–75.

BACKGROUND

Begin by reading some of the literature cited on the previous page. These sources will give you an understanding of both some of the current techniques used to manage acute pain and the issues or barriers that contribute to ineffective pain management.

The management of acute pain in British hospitals has long been criticised, but recent initiatives have done much to improve the situation. In this chapter, you will initially explore the concept of acute pain from the patients' viewpoint before considering some of the common interventions used to alleviate acute pain. You will be constantly considering the management of acute pain in terms of your own clinical experiences and the findings from research studies in this area. This sets the scene to provide a context before we explore, in greater detail, the strategies available to manage pain effectively.

Despite the advent of new technologies such as patient-controlled analgesia (PCA) and continuous epidural analgesia, the role of the ward nurse is crucial to the effective delivery of pain care. All too often, however, the most effective strategies are the simpler ones (McQuay et al., 1997). In the early 1990s, the American Agency for Health Care Policy and Research produced some excellent practice guidelines for the management of acute pain (AHCPR, 1992). There are now newer guidelines being produced regularly as health care takes on the philosophy of evidence-based practice. Excellent publications, such as those of McQuay and Moore (1998) and Carr and Goudas (1999), are also now available.

THE PATIENTS' PERSPECTIVE – EXPERIENCING ACUTE PAIN

Many patients in both hospital and the community continue to suffer unrelieved pain, and up to three-quarters of patients experience moderate to severe pain while in hospital (Royal College of Surgeons and College of Anaesthetists, 1990). A random sample of 5150 patients who had been recently discharged from hospital were interviewed, findings revealing that 61 per cent cited problems experienced in relation to pain management, and that 33 per cent of those suffering experienced pain all or most of the time (Bruster et al., 1994).

As we stated in the previous chapter, pain has been defined as 'an unpleasant sensory and emotional experience associated with actual or potential tissue damage, or described in terms of such damage' (IASP, 1986, p. 5216). Let us look at how the patient views pain. Before we do this, however, it is important to take a closer look at your ward, unit or community setting.

Time out   In a day, about how many people do you encounter who are experiencing acute pain?
Ask family or friends who have had an acute pain experience (surgery or some type of trauma) whether they were offered pain relief. How did they feel?

Most people have at one time or another experienced pain. Interestingly, many people put up with inadequate pain management because of their low expectations concerning pain relief: they may feel that it is an inevitable part of the situation (Carr and Thomas, 1997).

Donovan (1990) suggests that acute pain is usually associated with a specific event. We sometimes consider only trauma and surgical inter-

Activity

Select two patients and ask them to tell you about their pain. To do this, it is necessary to be fairly unstructured as you want them to talk as 'openly' as possible and give you plenty of information.

Sample questions are:

- Tell me about your pain.
- What helps your pain?
- What could the nurses do to make your pain better or help you to cope with it?

Each interview should take 10–20 minutes. Audiotaping it will save you having to take notes (but always ask the patient's permission first). Otherwise, write down as much as you can. Include your observations of the patient (facial expression, body language and so on).

vention to be the causes of acute pain, but what about other procedures that patients frequently undergo: radiology, dental treatment, venepuncture, drain removal, suturing and stitch removal? Madjar (1998) writes vividly about her interviews with burn patients and patients receiving chemotherapy. The book narrates the lived experience of pain inflicted in the context of prescribed medical treatment. It explores the pain from the perspective of the patients who endured it and of the nurses whose actions contributed.

Time out   Reflect on the findings from your interview.
              What are the implications for your practice?

Why treat acute pain?

While it is unethical to allow patients to suffer, it is also extremely detrimental to their recovery. When pain is acute and uncontrolled, the patient is unlikely to move, preferring to lie as still as possible to avoid inducing excruciating pain. This has several unwanted side-effects: respiratory function, for example, may be compromised, and coughing and deep breathing may be avoided, thus predisposing to chest infection.

In the past, we have underestimated the damage that pain may cause, and there is also evidence that unrelieved acute pain may develop into a chronic problem (Jayson, 1997). A prospective study on breast cancer patients explored whether the intensity of previous postoperative pain was a primary factor predisposing them to the development of chronic post-treatment pain. Ninety-three women were interviewed preoperatively and three times over the year following surgery. The results suggested that the amount of postoperative pain they experienced might play a role in the development of chronic pain (Tasmuth et al., 1996).

WHAT ARE ACUTE PAIN SERVICES?

The concept of the Acute Pain Service (APS) originated in the United States, led by an anaesthetist called Brian Ready in Seattle. It was to provide a template for development of services in the United Kingdom

(Ready *et al.*, 1988). A report from the Royal College of Surgeons and College of Anaesthetists (1990) concluded that the traditional methods of managing pain after surgery, for example opioid analgesia given intramuscularly, were inadequate and recommended that an APS be introduced into all major hospitals performing surgery in the United Kingdom. By 1995, 57 per cent of hospitals had an acute pain team (Windsor *et al.*, 1996), and this figure is probably gradually increasing.

The acute pain service or team usually comprises one or more anaesthetists, an acute pain clinical nurse specialist and a pharmacist. Some teams may also possess a clinical psychologist. The team is responsible for the day-to-day management of pain after surgery and trauma, and for ensuring that adequate monitoring is available for the pain-relieving technique chosen, for example epidural analgesia or PCA. Education features prominently, and many run in-service training on analgesic techniques as well as on pain-related topics. In many hospital wards, nurses now routinely care for patients receiving epidural analgesia, whereas a few years ago these patients would have been nursed in an intensive care unit. The teams also undertake research related to pain, and it is standard practice for them to audit the service continuously in order to evaluate the effectiveness of these initiatives.

Time out   Think about how the role of the ward nurse in managing pain has changed over the past 10 years.
Can you foresee any negative aspects?

The role of the ward nurse is critical to the success of the endeavours of the acute pain team, and it has been suggested that hospital nurses need further education to enable them to broaden their role in pain management (Mather and Ready, 1994). There is a concern that the role of ward nurses might be eroded as they see 'experts' taking responsibility for pain management (Notcutt, 1997). It is, therefore, essential that nurses are empowered to take responsibility for pain management and to adopt an active role in assessing pain and evaluating the effectiveness of interventions.

Activity

If ward nurses are to be 'empowered', how might this be done?

What is the role of the APS in your hospital?

Does the team see all patients with PCA and epidurals, or do the ward nurses only call the team if there are problems?

THE FUTURE OF ACUTE PAIN SERVICES

Despite the introduction of these teams in many hospitals across the United Kingdom, evidence suggests that some patients are still slipping through the net (Audit Commission, 1997). There is no doubt that the introduction of new pain technologies has done much to improve the quality of pain relief for many patients. Some see the natural development of acute pain teams into 'perioperative care' areas, where nutrition, fluid balance, the prevention of deep vein thrombosis, and mobilisation complement their role in the provision of analgesia (Jones, 1998). This is already happening in Copenhagen, and there is much discussion on the multimodal approach to improving recovery and preventing the unwanted side-effects of surgery (Kehlet, 1997).

All too often, health care professionals do not explore patients' views on their pain management but focus instead on pharmacological interventions. Strategies such as relaxation, distraction, information-giving, comfort (positioning) and presencing (being with the patient) can all contribute greatly to the reduction of pain or help patients to 'cope' with their pain. You may have found that the patients to whom you have spoken mentioned non-pharmacological strategies that helped their pain; we will cover some of these strategies later on in the chapter.

Time out Think about the interventions commonly used to manage acute pain in your area.
Make a list of these to review later.

In the next section, we will consider the pharmacological management of acute pain and consider some of the current methods of administration, such as PCA, as well as strategies to maximise analgesic administration. In addition to pharmacological interventions, it is important to complement these with non-pharmacological strategies.

PHARMACOLOGICAL APPROACHES TO PAIN MANAGEMENT

Analgesics are some of the most common 'over the counter' drugs (OTC), but knowledge is required for their optimal effectiveness. It is essential to teach patients how drugs work, their possible side-effects and how to avoid these. Although analgesics are generally prescribed by doctors within the hospital setting, the administration of analgesia to the patient is viewed as primarily a nursing role. It is, therefore, necessary that nurses are knowledgeable in pharmacology and are able to apply this knowledge critically to their practice.

Knowledge of analgesia in terms of dose, effectiveness, side-effects and how drugs can be combined to give balanced analgesia is the basis of good pain relief. There is no great myth or complexity to this – just clear understanding and confidence. Nurses also need to educate patients on analgesia: not only the side-effects, but also the rationale. Many patients (and health care staff) are reluctant to take analgesia, but a clear understanding of why it is important to be comfortable will encourage patients to accept pain relief and report its inadequacies.

Commonly used analgesics

We shall now cover some of the most commonly used analgesics, starting with those used in most households on a regular basis.

To indicate visually the various forms in which these drugs are available, we have used the following symbols:

Tablet	Injection	Liquid	Cream	Sublingual preparation	Effervescent solution	Suppository

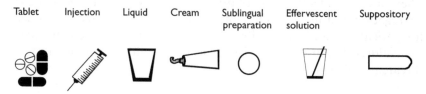

Analgesics for mild pain

Paracetamol

Most of us have used this drug at some time. It is useful for mild pain and can be used in combination with other drugs for mild to moderate pain. Paracetamol often considerably increases the effectiveness of other analgesics. For example, with codeine 60 mg, you need to give the drug to approximately 17 patients for one patient to achieve a 50 per cent relief of his or her pain score (the efficacy of analgesics being expressed as the number needed to treat (NNT) – the lower the number, the better). If 1g paracetamol is given with 60 mg codeine, the NNT is reduced to around 3. See McQuay et al. (1997) for further information on NNTs and analgesia.

Paracetamol is also useful for lowering the temperature. It is thought to work by predominantly inhibiting the body's synthesis of prostaglandin in the central nervous system, certain prostaglandins being known to be potent pain-producing substances.

Unlike non-steroidal anti-inflammatory drugs (NSAIDs), paracetamol does not appear to have a strong effect at the peripheral level so does not, therefore, produce gastric irritation and does not affect platelet function. Paracetamol is useful for non-inflammatory pain such as a headache but is not particularly good on its own for severe pain. It can be highly toxic if taken as an overdose, and, as it has a ceiling effect, there is no point in exceeding the recommended dose anyway.

Aspirin

Aspirin is also useful for mild pain, combining the properties of reducing both temperature and inflammation. Unfortunately, unlike paracetamol, it is very irritant to the stomach, and it can cause a severe asthmatic attack in about 5–10 per cent of patients who have developed adult-onset asthma. However, if an asthmatic patient has used aspirin in the past with no ill effect, it is safe to use it again. There are also plenty of alternatives. Aspirin acts to inhibit platelet aggregation and increase the clotting time so it is not recommended for patients on anticoagulation therapy. It is also not recommended for children because of the risk of Reye's syndrome, an acute, life-threatening illness.

Opioids and their use

Opioids come in a range of effectiveness from weak to strong. In their strongest form, they can be used as a first-line drug for pain of such severity that milder drugs are not expected to provide adequate relief. This is particularly the case following any painful surgery or trauma. Whether they are given in their strongest or their weakest form, they can also be combined with paracetamol, aspirin or another NSAID, especially when any of these drugs fails to provide adequate analgesia for acute pain on its own.

Although opioids can be very strong, they are best used for dull pain, that is, pain that travels to the spinal cord via the C fibres (see Chapter 1). Opioids act by binding to the opioid receptors principally distributed throughout the central nervous system, thereby modulating the transmission of pain impulses. Opioids are not effective for sharp incident pain, that is, pain transmitted via the A delta fibres. It is also true that only a very few chronic pain syndromes respond well to opioids. However, for severe pain following trauma or an operation, for an acutely painful medical condition, or for patients with cancer pain, they can provide powerful pain relief.

To simplify matters, we will just concentrate on the most commonly used opioids, starting with the weaker drugs: codeine, dihydrocodeine and dextropropoxyphene.

The weaker opioids

Codeine

This drug comes from the opium poppy and has been a mainstay of analgesia for many years. Recently, however, its efficacy versus side-effect profile has brought it and other weak opioids under increasing scrutiny (McQuay and Moore, 1998). It is biotransformed to morphine but is much less potent. It is usually given in doses of 30–60 mg; frequently as a combined preparation with paracetamol. Although doses above 90 mg may still be effective, the side-effects usually preclude amounts larger than this. Codeine can cause quite severe constipation and, when used for the first time, usually leaves people feeling drowsy and light-headed. The dose that can be bought over the counter in combined analgesic preparations is, however, very small – no more than 8 mg.

Dihydrocodeine

This is a derivative of codeine and is slightly more potent. Although the side-effects are the same as for codeine, it may cause more confusion and disorientation, especially in children and the elderly.

Dextropropoxyphene

This drug is quite weak: in a meta-analysis of studies, 65 mg given on its own appeared to provide less pain relief than 500 mg of paracetamol (McQuay and Moore, 1998). When 65 mg dextropropoxyphene is combined with 650 mg paracetamol as co-proxamol, it seems to perform about as well as 1000 mg paracetamol alone, but with greater side-effects. It is, however, still a much-loved preparation among the elderly and in the community. It is not recommended for anything other than mild to moderate pain and, with newer treatments now available, there is a growing need to assess its suitability for postoperative patients or those with any significant trauma (McQuay and Moore, 1998). Dextropropoxyphene appears to be slightly less constipating than the other two opioids mentioned above, but it still causes drowsiness and dizziness.

The following case history illustrates how even a small change in a drug regime can improve a patient's pain control.

case history

You have an elderly patient on your ward who has been taking co-proxamol for many years to control pain from an arthritic hip. He cannot tolerate NSAIDs as he has a past history of peptic ulcer disease. He has now been admitted to hospital for investigations of an unrelated condition but has found that his increased immobility and the anxiety of being in hospital are making his hip pain more difficult to control. What would you suggest?

Possible solution: As the co-proxamol that this man takes regularly contains only 325 mg paracetamol in each tablet, combined with a weak opioid, he might benefit from taking a combined analgesic that has 500 mg paracetamol per tablet with either 8 mg codeine (co-codamol) or 10 mg dihydrocodeine (co-dydramol) rather than dextropropoxyphene. If this still fails to control your patient's pain adequately, one of the combined preparations containing 30 mg codeine plus 500 mg paracetamol per tablet may be helpful. Alternatively, while your patient is in hospital, and provided that his pain still responds to opioids, it might be useful to try substituting all the weak opioids for a small regular dose of oral morphine in either tablet or syrup form.

There are newer and safer oral NSAIDs becoming available all the time; a trial of a short course of one of these, with close monitoring for any adverse side-effects, might be appropriate. Many NSAIDs are also available as topical preparations, and these may be well worth a trial: topical NSAIDs are not associated with the gastrointestinal adverse effects that are seen with the same drugs taken orally (Evans *et al.*, 1995). Remember also to include non-pharmacological strategies, which will be covered briefly at the end of this chapter.

Stronger opioids

Morphine

Morphine, like codeine, has its origins in the opium poppy. Its powerful effects have been known for a very long time: there is in fact evidence that these poppies have been cultivated since the third century BC.

Although by no means an ideal drug, or one that will work for all types of pain, morphine still remains the so-called 'gold standard' by which all other pain-relieving drugs are judged. In the authors' experience, it is often underused for moderate to severe acute pain. It is frequently observed that a dose of oral morphine, titrated to the patient's response, will produce rapid and adequate analgesia with fewer side-effects than a large dose of a weaker opioid. We have also found that oral morphine syrup is particularly useful for children, especially if a policy of 'no intramuscular analgesia' is to be encouraged. Surprisingly few studies have been conducted on the use of oral morphine syrup, and it could be that a resistance to the extensive use of this preparation is the result of myth and misconception rather than of well-conducted trials that form the basis of evidence-based practice.

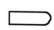

Diamorphine

Although this drug is converted in the body to morphine, it is said to have a faster onset of action with a shorter duration of effect. It can be dissolved in a very small quantity of water or saline, which is beneficial for patients needing a continuous subcutaneous infusion.

For example, 60 mg diamorphine in 10 ml normal saline attached to a small portable infusion pump can be delivered over 24 hours.

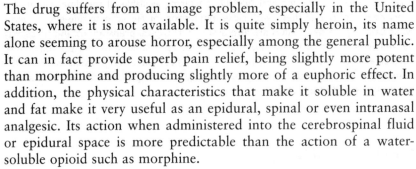

The drug suffers from an image problem, especially in the United States, where it is not available. It is quite simply heroin, its name alone seeming to arouse horror, especially among the general public. It can in fact provide superb pain relief, being slightly more potent than morphine and producing slightly more of a euphoric effect. In addition, the physical characteristics that make it soluble in water and fat make it very useful as an epidural, spinal or even intranasal analgesic. Its action when administered into the cerebrospinal fluid or epidural space is more predictable than the action of a water-soluble opioid such as morphine.

Methadone

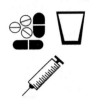

In the United Kingdom, methadone is used to treat drug addicts and is rarely used to control acute pain. It is a powerful pain killer, about as potent as morphine, but lasts longer and can, when used regularly, accumulate, causing problems. It is, however, occasionally useful when morphine is not providing adequate analgesia.

Pethidine

Pethidine is only about one-tenth as potent as morphine, being even weaker when given by mouth. It also has a very short duration of action: somewhere between 1 and 3 hours. The other problem is its metabolite norpethidine, which can accumulate when large doses of the drug are given or it is used for longer than a few days. Norpethidine is toxic and may cause convulsions.

Pethidine has, however, some advantages. Certain patients prefer it, and it is always useful to be able to offer an alternative if a patient has had a bad experience with morphine. It has also been one of the drugs of choice for renal or biliary colic. However, the old idea that pethidine is better than other opioids as a treatment for colicky pain, especially biliary and renal colic, is being seriously questioned (Nagle and McQuay, 1990; McQuay, 1999). A further note of caution is that this drug can be dangerous if given to a patient taking a monoamine oxidase inhibitor; the combination has been known to send patients spiralling into a hypertensive crisis.

Phenazocine

This is a strong synthetic opioid that was first developed in the 1950s and has been largely forgotten. Phenazocine is now available only in tablet form, but it has an extremely useful property in that it is very effective when taken sublingually, being in fact as effective as morphine. This means that it can be taken by patients who are not able to tolerate oral medication. Although there is very little literature available on this drug, it has been reported to cause less nausea and vomiting (Economou *et al.*, 1971) and sedation (Blair, 1967) than morphine; this has certainly been the authors' experience. It is time perhaps to conduct further studies into this potentially very useful yet little used drug.

Other opioids

There are two other drugs that are probably worth mentioning here: nalbuphine (Nubain), which is often used by ambulance staff, and the still quite popular buprenorphine (Temgesic). These differ from the other opioids in the way in which they work. The opioids previously discussed are what are termed pure agonists – they bind firmly to opioid receptors on the nerve membrane – but nalbuphine and buprenorphine do not act in quite this way.

Nalbuphine

Nalbuphine (Nubain) is different as it is an antagonist at one opioid receptor, the mu, but acts as an agonist at the kappa receptor. The continued agonist–antagonist action means that there is a ceiling effect for both analgesia and side-effects. This limits the drug's effect but does so in safety. The drug does not come under the same administration and storage controls as the opioids previously mentioned. Because of these factors, it is widely used by ambulance staff for patients on their way to accident and emergency (A&E) departments. It is only available for parenteral administration, which limits its use elsewhere. Because it acts as an agonist/antagonist, this drug can become an antagonist when another pure agonist is administered. If you wish, return briefly to Chapter 1 to refresh your memory on the physiology surrounding agonists and antagonists before answering the following question.

Nalbuphine can act either as an agonist (giving pain relief) or an antagonist (blocking the receptors) when a pure agonist is administered. In hospital, the A&E staff may want to give a powerful opioid to relieve pain. If the drug of choice is a pure agonist (for example, morphine) and some Nalbuphine still remains in the patient's system, effective pain relief might not be achieved as the Nalbuphine starts to block the receptors in the presence of the agonist. How does your local A&E department manage pain?

Buprenorphine

Buprenorphine (Temgesic) is a partial agonist and is about 50 times more potent than morphine. The fact that it is longlasting (acting for about 8–10 hours) and also comes as a sublingual preparation makes it appealing. It is also supposed to cause less physical dependence. Interestingly, however, patients seem to either love it or hate it, those who hate it complaining of excessive nausea and light-headedness.

Naloxone

Naloxone (Narcan) has no other action than to reverse the effects of opioids. It is, therefore, only ever used to reverse an opioid overdose. Its administration often needs to be repeated, as the opioid action will return within about half an hour, and it will not necessarily reverse a partial agonist such as buprenorphine. Used in small doses, that is, 0.2 µg intramuscularly, it is also excellent for reversing an opioid-induced urinary retention; it has often removed the need to catheterise a patient, much to his or her relief. In the same small dose, it can be used to treat an opioid-induced itch that does not respond to a dose of antihistamine.

For a useful and provocative discourse on opioids, see McQuay (1999). Although this article focuses primarily on chronic and cancer pain, many of the principles apply also to acute pain.

Time out   Think of a patient who has been taking an opioid.
Was there any reason indicated for why he or she was taking that
particular drug?
If you get the chance, ask the prescribing doctor why he chose it.
You will unfortunately often find that it was a prescribing habit
rather than an evidence-based decision or the result of an
evaluation of patient response.

Non-steroidal anti-inflammatory agents

Non-steroidal anti-inflammatory agents (NSAIDs) is a term for a large group of drugs that reduce inflammation. Most of them produce some analgesia after just one dose, but they are usually best given regularly to reduce any swelling, muscle tenderness or joint stiffness. Like aspirin and paracetamol, these drugs affect the body's synthesis of prostaglandin, but the NSAIDs do this mostly at the site of tissue damage. They are very good for mild to moderate pain and will some-times be useful for even quite severe pain. They are also of benefit when given with opioid analgesics, providing additional analgesia and reducing the need for a large dose of opioid. For NSAIDs, there is a ceiling effect so exceeding the recommended dose will not achieve better analgesia and could greatly increase the risk of potentially dangerous side-effects. In some recent studies, NSAIDs provided pain relief equivalent to or even better than 10 mg intramuscular morphine (McQuay and Moore, 1998).

Which NSAID?

There is a vast range of these drugs, which can be given in a variety of ways. If a patient taking an NSAID obtains only a disappointing relief of his or her pain, it is often worthwhile changing to another NSAID from a different chemical class. Two types of NSAID must, however, never be given together as this may result in serious side-effects.

Below are listed some popular NSAIDs divided into their chemically related groups:

Group 1	Group 2	Group 3	Group 4	Group 5
Ibuprofen	Diclofenac	Indomethacin	Piroxicam	Mefenamic
Naproxen	Ketorolac			Acid

65

Although NSAIDs are usually very effective, especially following injury or surgery, they can have some particularly serious side-effects that limit their use. Many of these side-effects are seen with long-term use so the use of NSAIDs for only a few days is relatively safe. A new type of NSAID described as COX-2 specific is currently becoming available, which, because of its selective action, could prove to be safer, even when given to patients traditionally contraindicated to receive NSAIDs (Needleman and Isakson, 1998).

For postoperative patients, it has been argued that the risks associated with the side-effects of NSAIDs are sometimes overemphasised. Provided that they are prescribed with care, and nurses are aware of what to look for in patients who may be adversely affected by the drugs, the majority of patients can benefit from the NSAIDs' pain-relieving properties, particularly those patients experiencing excessive prostaglandin release following surgery.

Excellent guidelines on the use of NSAIDS are available from the Royal College of Anaesthetists (1998).

Entonox

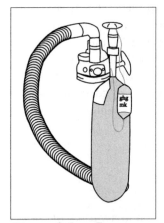

Figure 3.1   Entonox delivery apparatus

Entonox, a 50 per cent mixture of oxygen and nitrous oxide, is often overlooked when trying to control acute pain, even though it can be very safe and effective. Nitrous oxide is an analgesic gas that has a rapid onset and is excreted rapidly from the body when no longer inhaled. It is able to act so quickly because the tiny molecules cross the capillary walls in the lungs straight into the bloodstream.

As patients hold the mask themselves, Entonox can be considered to be a form of PCA, that is, the patient controls how much gas he or she receives. Entonox is available in portable cylinders for bedside use that comprise a length of tubing with a mask or mouthpiece and a patient demand valve (Figure 3.1). The gas is odourless and colourless, the smell associated with it, which can upset some patients, usually arising from the mask; this can be overcome by using a mouthpiece. When used properly via a close-fitting mask or mouthpiece held in place for at least 1 minute, analgesia can be maintained, but the effects wear off very quickly once the gas is no longer being inhaled. For short painful procedures such as catheterisation, dressing changes, mobilising painful joints and so on, the gas can provide very good pain relief, especially when used in combination with other analgesics. It has been used extensively for labour pain.

Entonox has proved very valuable for ambulance crews and in A&E, where it is often used to provide pain relief for the simple suturing of wounds and other painful procedures. The gas can even be used to reduce a dislocated finger or a shoulder provided that the associated muscle spasm is not severe. The gas is extremely safe to use as there is no drop in blood pressure or serious drop in level of consciousness, although some patients may become drowsy, dizzy or even feel sick. There are a small group of patients who should not receive Entonox. Because nitrous oxide rapidly diffuses into air-filled spaces, it must not be given to patients for whom this may cause problems:

- if pneumothorax is suspected or shown
- cases of bowel obstruction
- those with severe head injury
- decompression sickness.

Maximising the analgesic prescription

Evidence suggests that there are many missed opportunities, leading to prescribed analgesia not being as potentially effective as it could be (Griepp, 1992; Carr and Thomas, 1997; Brockopp et al., 1998). It is imperative that the nurse takes an active role to ensure that the patient obtains the maximum benefit from the analgesia. The nurse is often faced with an array of 'PRN' analgesics, presenting an ideal opportunity to ensure that the analgesia selected offers 'balanced analgesia' or multimodal pain treatment (Dahl et al., 1990), the premise being that total pain relief cannot be achieved through the use of a single drug or method without the risk of significant adverse effects. Combining different drugs, such as an NSAID and a centrally acting drug (such as an opioid), offers greater potential pain relief than when the agents are used individually. There is no need to limit this to pharmacological approaches as combining analgesia and non-pharmacological interventions can optimise pain control by exploiting the multidimensional nature of pain.

The following are examples of some of the potential opportunities to maximise analgesic effectiveness:

- Check the prescription and ensure that the dose and the time interval between doses are correct. Research suggests that doctors frequently underprescribe analgesia and overestimate the dose duration.

- When the dose of analgesia is prescribed as a variable amount, for example 10–20 mg, titrate the analgesia against the pain rather than always giving the smallest amount possible.

- Avoid abrupt transitions from parental opioids to non-opioids (Smith, 1998). The World Health Organization's (WHO, 1996) analgesic ladder (Figure 3.2) is useful used in reverse to guide analgesic strengths.

- Educate patients about their analgesia and why they should be comfortable, for example to enable them to mobilise and prevent complications. This will make them more likely to be open about their pain and to accept analgesia.

- If an opioid has been prescribed, request that an antiemetic and laxative also be ordered, and use these proactively.

- Around-the-clock dosing is more effective than traditional PRN regimes; give analgesia before the pain returns rather than after it has done so.

- Fear of respiratory depression and addiction are often reasons why health care professionals are reluctant to prescribe and administer opioids. Research indicates these fears are unfounded as fewer than

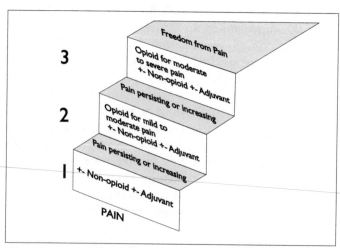

Figure 3.2 World Health Organization pain ladder (Reproduced with permission from WHO, 1996)

1 per cent of patients suffer these unwanted side-effects (Friedman, 1990). Every opportunity should be taken to dispel these myths.

Activity

For each of the previous statements, consider the practices and attitudes in your own clinical environment.

Make notes on your observations. For example, review the prescription charts and record how many analgesics are prescribed, along with the correct duration of dose.

case history

John Little is a 19-year-old man who was admitted to your ward following a compound fracture of his tibia and fibula. He was given pethidine 100 mg intramuscularly in the A&E department soon after his arrival there. The pethidine worked very well, but John found that it was beginning to wear off after about an hour. He was told he would be given more pain relief when he was admitted to a trauma ward. Because of the general activity level both in A&E and on the ward, 3 hours elapsed between John's first dose of pethidine and the next, during which time he became quite distressed with the pain. A second dose of pethidine 100 mg intramuscularly was administered on the ward, but the analgesia that this provided was not evaluated, and John did not have his pain assessed on a regular basis. The ward was so busy that John only asked for further analgesia when he could stand the pain no longer. Again, because of the workload, this usually involved a 30-minute delay between his request for urgent pain relief and its being administered.

John finds his pain is being very poorly controlled and complains to his family when they come to visit. This is then conveyed to the nurses, who feel a bit aggrieved because they feel that John should have let them know earlier that he was in such pain. John, of course, was trying to hide his pain because he was concerned that the nurses were so busy, he felt that his pain had to be really bad for him to trouble them.

Problems illustrated:

- John's pain is not being assessed properly and the effect of the pethidine evaluated. If this had been done, it would have been known that he was obtaining only 1 hour's pain relief.

- Regular assessment would have enabled analgesia to be administered before the pain became intolerable.

- Early assessment would have raised the question of whether pethidine was appropriate, its duration of action for John being only about 1 hour.

- The original dose was given intramuscularly to establish analgesia rapidly. However, John is fully able to tolerate oral medication, and this should have been prescribed for ongoing medication.

- Assessment would have not only established that pethidine was too short acting, but would have also shown that John was going to need regular medication for at least the first 24–48 hours.

- An NSAID, which could have been particularly useful for this bone trauma pain, was not prescribed. John has no contraindications to NSAIDs.

Possible solutions:

- Regular and ongoing pain assessment would have stopped this situation arising: half-hourly to hourly when initiating analgesia, and then 4-hourly to establish effective ongoing pain relief.

- Any problems arising would be detected early. A short-acting intramuscular opioid such as pethidine could be replaced with a regular, longer-acting drug such as oral morphine syrup as necessary.

- The use of a regular NSAID such as diclofenac, commenced in A&E, could well have established analgesia effectively enough to omit or reduce the need for opioids altogether.

- The regular administration of effective analgesia titrated to the patient's needs and administered during the routine drug round would have been far less distressing for John and would also have reduced the nursing workload.

Patient-controlled analgesia

PCA is a method of pain control that has been shown to provide more effective pain relief than traditional intramuscular analgesia (Ballantyne *et al.*, 1993). PCA involves patient control of a pump to self-administer analgesia via an intravenous or subcutaneous cannula. The pump is preprogrammed to deliver a small bolus dose of analgesia when the patient presses the button, but a 'lock-out' period prevents the patient receiving further doses should he or she press again within, for example, 5 minutes.

Several advantages exist for patients. PCA enables them to receive analgesia when they need it as they do not have to ask a nurse or wait for the nurse to prepare the analgesia. It also avoids the unwanted peaks (leading to sedation, nausea and so on) and troughs (pain) associated with the larger doses used in intramuscular administration. The patient administers small doses, which ensure that the plasma concentration can be kept within a therapeutic level.

Activity

If your ward is currently using PCA, what level of involvement do you have with it?

What are the advantages for the patient (ask someone who has used it) and what do staff think of PCA? What are the advantages and disadvantages for them?

Compare your findings with those of Thomas (1993).

Research on PCA is very interesting, revealing quite contradictory findings. PCA may not work for all patients as some people do not feel comfortable being responsible for the administration of their own analgesia (Thomas and Rose, 1993). Consider the wide variety of clinical settings that have used PCA and discuss some of the patient variables, such as locus of control and coping style, that may affect the efficacy of PCA. Taylor *et al.* (1996) interviewed patients about using PCA and found negative and positive evaluations, the negative ones including nausea and inadequate analgesia. It has been found, by Koh and Thomas (1994), that PCA saves nursing time but that patients receiving PCA are no more satisfied than those receiving traditional intramuscular analgesia. A useful source of information on PCA is Welchew (1995).

Epidural analgesia

Epidural analgesia is becoming increasingly popular as a method of providing effective pain relief. It is often used postoperatively and during labour. The epidural space is located between the dura mater and the spinal canal. A fine catheter is inserted into the epidural space, between the vertebrae, allowing the delivery of analgesics.

Opioid drugs can be given in small quantities as they diffuse through the dura mater, binding to opioid receptors in the spinal cord and thus producing analgesia. Local anaesthetic agents such as bupivacaine can also be used, exerting their action by anaesthetising the nerves that leave the spinal cord; this numbs pain in the area supplied by these nerves, for example abdominal wall muscle.

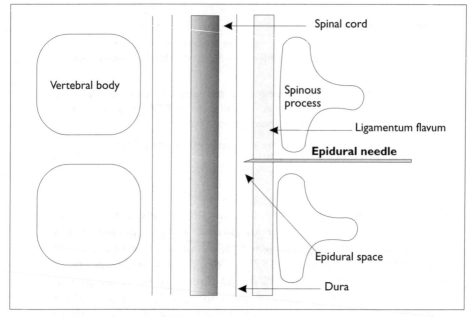

Figure 3.3 Location of the needle in the epidural space through which a catheter is threaded to enable continuous drug administration

Jaques (1994) provides an excellent paper outlining the physiology, nursing care and possible complications associated with this method and a review of the possible benefits of epidural analgesia is contained in Spencer et al. (1995).

NON-PHARMACOLOGICAL APPROACHES TO ACUTE PAIN MANAGEMENT

Pain is a multidimensional phenomenon and, as we have already explored (through Gate Control Theory; see Chapter 1), has physical, emotional and cognitive components. It is essential then that effective pain interventions reflect this phenomenon and that pharmacological interventions are complemented by non-pharmacological approaches administered simultaneously. Many of the interventions used in the management of chronic pain are very helpful in the management of acute pain too. The reader is referred to Chapter 4 for more information, as well as to an excellent article by Stevenson (1995).

The following interventions have been selected as they are becoming more widely used in acute pain, but this is only an introduction to a fascinating field of management.

Transcutanous electrical nerve stimulation

Transcutaneous electrical nerve stimulation (TENS) is a non-invasive method for the relief of both acute and chronic pain. The apparatus consists of a small electrical pulse generator, the size of a personal stereo, with two or four electrodes that are placed on the skin. It is battery powered, and the electrical impulse discharged can be altered in intensity, duration and frequency for each individual. It is suggested that the electrical stimulation excites the larger-diameter A beta fibres and closes the 'gate', as well as stimulating the release of endorphins (Hargreaves and Lander, 1989). The TENS machine can easily be worn beneath the clothes and does not restrict mobility, which allows the patient to continue normal activities such as work or gardening.

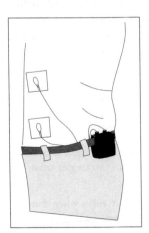

Figure 3.4   A TENS machine attached to a patient's belt with the electrodes applied to the right side of his back

Activity

Find out where you might obtain a TENS machine in your hospital and/or community.

Identify how to meet your own learning needs so that you could recommend it to a patient or friend and teach them how to use it. Speak to someone who has used a machine and find out how they use it for pain relief.

MASSAGE

As with the TENS machine, it is thought that, by stimulating the skin, the large-diameter A beta fibres can be activated, which then close the 'gate' and prevent pain impulses from A delta and C fibres reaching the central nervous system. Gentle firm stroking of the foot, hand or arm is often a very effective relaxation intervention for pain relief and can easily be used while waiting for analgesia to take effect, during a procedure or while washing, for example. Family and friends often feel helpless in relieving the suffering of pain, but simple massage or gentle stroking can bring pain relief and also help them to feel needed.

Relaxation

Psychological strategies are widely used for the reduction of distress and anxiety by reducing muscle tension, encouraging an inner sense of calm and diminishing the activity of the autonomic nervous system. They should be used in addition to pharmacological interventions. Pain often produces anxiety, which in turn produces muscle tension and more pain. Breaking the cycle is an important way of reducing the pain or helping the person to cope with his or her pain.

Activity

The next time you are with patients who have been experiencing pain, ask them whether they find any strategies other than medication useful.

Ask them what they do to help themselves relax when they feel tense.

Make notes on this and on the effectiveness of any of the strategies they mention.

Deep breathing strategies such as counting up to 10 slowly and then back again as one exhales is a method of focusing on breathing and reducing tension and anxiety. Music can be used as a relaxation or distraction strategy in pain management. A detailed review of studies on the effects of relaxation and music on postoperative pain concluded that they reduced the pain, especially the affective (emotional) component (Good, 1996). Using a personal stereo, the volume can be increased or decreased in response to the pain. Patients can be encouraged to bring in their favourite music. Watching an interesting programme on the television, or listening to the radio, when uncomfortable procedures are taking place may aid relaxation.

Distraction

Distraction is a strategy that allows one's mind to focus on pleasant stimuli rather than on the pain or negative emotions (McCaffery and Beebe, 1994). Distraction strategies are often routinely used by patients who experience chronic pain; they can range from watching television and reading a book, to listening to music or going for a walk. Most people have developed their own distraction activities to help them to cope with pain, but when they arrive in hospital they might feel unable, or even forget, to use some of these useful techniques.

Activity

Ask four patients whether they use anything to distract themselves from pain when they are at home.

Are these currently being used while they are in hospital?

If not, how could they be incorporated into their care?

Comfort

Comfort is often forgotten as an actual intervention for pain control and can easily be overlooked. It is important to note here that these strategies may be particularly helpful with people who have learning disabilities or senile dementia. The inability to express one's pain must only contribute to the fear and dread of its getting worse. Comfort strategies can include positioning, the presence of family and friends, and the skilled companionship of nursing staff.

Skilled companionship

Nurses may avoid patients who are experiencing pain if they feel that there is nothing they can do or if it makes them feel awkward and uncomfortable. When pain is distressing, the close company of another person can help the sufferer to cope with the experience. Nurses can stay with the person and just be there for them. When nurses have stayed with patients at this time, they talk about the nurse 'knowing what I was going through' or say, 'I just knew that they were there and it helped me cope.' Holding the person, letting him or her talk and just sitting quietly are all important actions that should be part of the rich repertoire of nursing care. We should not fear another's pain or suffering but allow ourselves to enter their world and be there for them.

Activity

Look around your ward or department. Do we make it easy for patients to use any of these non-pharmacological strategies?

Can patients see outside to watch the sky and trees?

Are there televisions and radios available, or can their relatives bring them in?

Are there telephones by the beds so that patients may talk to their friends and relatives?

Are visiting times fairly generous?

Do you have enough skilled staff to be able to ensure comfort and skilled companionship?

Some of these things may not seem terribly relevant, but if you have pain that is difficult to control, access to some or all of the above can make a significant difference. If patients are being nursed in a far from ideal environment, and away from their home comforts, we should as nurses be able to articulate the benefits of some of these far from obvious pain-relieving strategies. Patient studies often cite the more esoteric as being of great value, but we lose sight of this in the hubbub of a district general hospital. Palliative care units, however, have been very successful in emphasising the benefits of environment, comfort and distraction.

CONCLUSION

This section has encouraged you critically to reflect on the current management of acute pain. It has utilised pharmacological and non-pharmacological strategies that reflect the multidimensional nature of pain in order to plan effective pain interventions. In practice, the approach to acute pain management might incorporate only pharmacological interventions, and it is essential to consider broader approaches. By reflecting on your own practice and that of your colleagues, it is possible to broaden the approaches being used. Encompassing the perspective of the patient will help to facilitate effective intervention and improve patient care.

It should be considered that the poor or inappropriate management of acute pain could well lead to the development of chronic benign pain. This is particularly the case with chronic low back pain, which will be covered in more depth in Chapter 4. Chronic low back pain was recognised as one of the most common and costly health problems in Western societies in the late twentieth century (Linton, 1994), even more alarming perhaps when one considers the statement by Waddell (1992) that most chronic back pain is the iatrogenic consequence of inappropriate medical advice. This is undoubtedly food for thought as we attempt to relieve acute pain effectively.

After a break, try the multiple-choice questionnaire below in order to self-assess your understanding so far.

Suggested further reading

Carr, E.C.J. (1990) Postoperative pain patients' expectations and experiences. *Journal of Advanced Nursing,* **15**: 89–100.

Good, M. (1996) Effects of relaxation and music on postoperative pain: a review. *Journal of Advanced Nursing,* **24**: 905–14.

Harmer, M., Davies, K.A. and Lunn, J.N. (1995) A survey of acute pain services in the United Kingdom. *British Medical Journal,* **311**: 360–1.

Hasking, J. and Welchen, E. (1985) *Postoperative Pain: Understanding its Nature and How To Treat It,* London, Faber and Faber.

Jurf, J.B. and Nirschl, A.L. (1993) Acute postoperative pain management: a comprehensive review and update. *Critical Care Nursing Quarterly,* 16(1): 8–25.

Justins, D.M. and Richardson, P.H. (1991) Clinical management of acute pain. *British Medical Journal,* 47: 561–83.

Park, G. and Fulton, B. (1991) *The Management of Acute Pain,* Oxford, Oxford Medical Publications.

Shipton, E.A. (1993) *Pain Acute and Chronic,* Johannesburg, Witwatersrand University Press.

Stevenson, C. (1995) Non-pharmacological aspects of acute pain management, *Complementary Therapies in Nursing and Midwifery,* 1: 77–84.

Managing Acute Pain

MULTIPLE-CHOICE QUESTIONNAIRE

1. Which of the following would you not associate with acute pain?

   a. Radiological procedures ☐
   b. Dental treatment ☐
   c. Trauma ☐
   d. Migraine ☐

2. Which of the following is a pain-producing substance that is blocked by treatment with NSAIDs?

   a. Prostaglandin ☐
   b. Prothrombin ☐
   c. Prostacyclin ☐
   d. Prolactin ☐

3. Which of the following is particularly useful for treating postoperative pain?

   a. Paracetamol ☐
   b. Codeine ☐
   c. NSAIDs ☐
   d. Dextropropoxyphene ☐

4. How are opioids thought to relieve pain?

   a. By reducing inflammation ☐
   b. By acting at the site of tissue damage ☐
   c. By blocking pain signals in the central nervous system ☐
   d. By making the patient sleep ☐

MULTIPLE-CHOICE QUESTIONNAIRE (cont'd)

5. Which of the following is not a common side-effect of opioids?

   a. Sedation ☐

   b. Nausea and vomiting ☐

   c. Constipation ☐

   d. Respiratory depression ☐

6. Which is the safest route by which to administer a titrated dose of opioid?

   a. Orally ☐

   b. Intramuscularly ☐

   c. Intravenously ☐

   d. Rectally ☐

7. Which statement accurately describes how TENS works?

   a. It distracts the patient from thinking about their pain ☐

   b. It works by exciting the nerve fibres and opening the pain gate ☐

   c. It stimulates the release of prostaglandins ☐

   d. It excites the A beta fibres and closes the pain gate ☐

8. Which of the following describes distraction?

   a. Thinking of a nice holiday and imagining that you are there ☐

   b. Slowly counting to 10 while breathing in, and then slowly exhaling ☐

   c. Watching television ☐

   d. Listening to a piano concerto by Brahms ☐

9. Who is critical to the success of an acute pain team?

   a. The anaesthetist ☐

   b. The acute pain sister/charge nurse ☐

   c. The ward nurse ☐

   d. The house officer ☐

10. Which statement would reflect a physical and psychological approach to the management of pain?

   a. PCA and imagery ☐

   b. Music and deep breathing ☐

   c. Regular NSAIDs and relaxation ☐

   d. Relaxation and paracetamol ☐

ANSWERS FOR THE MULTIPLE-CHOICE QUESTIONNAIRE

1. **d. Migraine**; headaches can be severe in intensity, but because they usually occur repeatedly over time, they are classified as being chronic. Radiological procedures may cause acute pain, for example when positioning a fractured limb, or pain of short duration, as with drain removal, which can result in clinicians failing actively to manage the pain.

2. **a. Prostaglandin E** is the end-product of a chain of chemical events that results once tissue damage has occurred. It is known to increase the activity of the nerves conducting pain impulses and therefore exacerbates the pain. Prothrombin is an inactive substance in blood plasma that is the precursor of thrombin, which clots the blood. Prostacyclin is a type of prostaglandin produced by the endothelial lining of the blood vessels; it inhibits platelet aggregation, thus reducing the blood clotting time. Prolactin is the pituitary hormone that initiates lactation.

3. **c. NSAIDs**; tissue damage following surgery results in a prostaglandin release.

4. **c. By blocking pain signals in the central nervous system**; NSAIDs reduce inflammation and also act at the site of tissue damage. Opioids can make patients feel sleepy, but this is incidental to their pain-relieving properties.

5. **d. Respiratory depression** is quite unusual when opioids are used correctly: it is very rare for opioids to induce respiratory depression once a patient has taken opioids for a few days. Sedation is quite common when opioids are used for the first time. Nausea and vomiting affect about 30 per cent of opioids users during the first few days of use, and constipation causes potential problems for the majority of opioid users.

6. **c. Intravenously**; this route is the safest as the onset of action is at less than 1 minute, and the peak effect (including unwanted side-effects) can usually be seen after 7 minutes. With oral administration, the onset of action can be anywhere between 5 minutes and 1 hour. Uptake from intramuscular injection is also variable (5–70 minutes), also being influenced by variables such as hydration, cold and hypotension.

7. **d. It excites the A beta fibres and closes the pain gate**; thus reducing the perception of pain. It is suggested that it may also encourage the release of endorphins.

8. **c. Watching television** is a distraction as it channels thoughts away from the pain. Thinking back to a nice holiday is termed 'imagery' and is a cognitive strategy (that is, it modifies thought processes) used in the management of pain. Distraction and imagery are both cognitive strategies. Deep breathing and listening to a relaxing piece of music are both behavioural strategies that modify the physiological reaction to pain.

9. **c. The ward nurse** needs to be empowered to take responsibility for pain management. This will include receiving further education for the role.

10. **a. PCA and imagery**; music and deep breathing are both behavioural strategies. Paracetamol, NSAIDs and relaxation are physical and behavioural approaches.

4

Managing chronic pain

LEARNING OUTCOMES

On completion of this chapter the student will be able to:

- Review the psychological, behavioural and physical strategies used in the management of chronic pain

- Critically discuss professional collaboration in the holistic management of the person experiencing pain

- Analyse practices for managing chronic pain in his or her own clinical area and identify methods of influencing change

---

INDICATIVE READING

Ashburn, M.A. and Staats P.S. (1999) Management of chronic pain. *Lancet,* **353**: 1865–9.

Cailliet, R. (1993) *Pain Mechanisms and Management.* Philadelphia, F.A. Davis. (See Chapter 9.)

Charlton, J.E. (1998) Pain management: training and education issues. In Carter, B. (ed.) *Perspectives on Pain: Mapping the Territory,* London, Arnold.

Diamond, A.W. and Coniam, S.W. (1993) *The Management of Chronic Pain,* Oxford, Oxford University Press.

Janelli, K. (1995) A comparative study of patients' and nurses' perceptions of pain relief. *International Journal of Palliative Nursing,* 1(2): 74–80.

Latham, J. (1993) Chronic pain, In Carroll, D. and Bowsher, D. (eds) *Pain Management and Nursing Care,* Oxford, Butterworth-Heinnemann, Chapter 6.

Potter, R.G. (1998) The prevention of chronic pain. In Carter, B. (ed.) *Perspectives on Pain, Mapping the Territory,* London, Arnold.

Sofaer, B. (1998) Counselling in the management of pain. In Carter, B. (ed.) *Perspectives on Pain; Mapping the Territory,* London, Arnold.

BACKGROUND

Begin by reading some of the literature cited in the indicative reading section above. This will provide an understanding both of some of the current interventions for the management of chronic pain and the issues and barriers that contribute to ineffective pain management. In the United States, the Agency for Health Care Policy and Research has produced excellent practice guidelines for the management of pain, and the reader is referred to the publication on cancer pain (Jacox *et al.*, 1994).

Chronic pain has been defined as pain that lasts continuously or inter- mittently for 3 months or more (IASP, 1986). Increased research over the past 5–10 years is, however, bringing this definition into question. For example, Waddell (1992) suggests that acute back pain, if treated inappropriately, can become chronic within days of its onset as a result of muscle wasting and loss of bone density. Potter (1998) also suggests that 3 months is too long a period defining acute pain as lasting less than 4 weeks.

Chronic pain can be further categorised as being either malignant or non-malignant. It is important to distinguish between the two as the approach to treatment is different. Chronic non-malignant pain (for example, arthritis) is persistent and has no end-point. McCaffery and Beebe (1989, p. 232) define it as:

> pain that has lasted 6 months or longer, is ongoing on a daily basis, is due to non-threatening causes, has not responded to currently available treat- ment methods, and may continue for the remainder of the patient's life.

The philosophy of treatment often focuses on helping patients to take responsibility for their pain and helping them to cope with it using a variety of stategies. Reducing the consumption of analgesia and teaching the patient coping strategies are common goals of treatment. In contrast, chronic malignant pain may have an end-point, treatment approaches including analgesia that is given in sufficient amount to relieve the pain, as well as other strategies reflecting the multi- dimensional nature of pain, for example relaxation and cutaneous stimulation.

Given the different approaches to the two types of chronic pain, this chapter will primarily consider chronic non-malignant pain, although many of the non-pharmacological approaches are equally helpful for chronic malignant pain. The reader is referred to Richardson (1997) for an informative discussion on cancer pain and its management. The following section explores chronic pain from the patient's perspective and considers some of the pharmacological and non-pharmacological interventions. Finally, the importance of professional collaboration is explored.

WHAT IS CHRONIC NON-MALIGNANT PAIN?

It is helpful to think about what types of disease might generate chronic pain. The obvious one is arthritis, but there are many others. Diabetes can lead to peripheral neuropathy, which can be painful. Any form of ischaemia (angina or intermittent claudication, for example) also generates pain, which can become a part of everyday life. Chronic obstructive airways disease can cause chest pain. Low back pain is particularly prevalent and has far reaching effects on a person's life.

Activity

Think of some more causes of chronic non-malignant pain.

Ask people whether they experience continuous pain.

An analysis of 1000 consultations in general practice revealed that 11.3 per cent were for a pain of more than 3 months' duration (Potter, 1990). Chronic low back pain is a major cause of personal suffering and financial burden, and has even been termed an 'epidemic' (Potter, 1998).

THE PATIENT'S PERSPECTIVE – EXPERIENCING CHRONIC PAIN

Let us now explore pain from the patient's perspective. Before we do this, however, take a close look around your clinical environment. How many patients (as a percentage) are experiencing chronic pain? Bear in mind they may also have acute pain. It would be helpful to explore their pain in greater depth, as in the following activity.

Activity

Select two patients within your clinical area who suffer from a chronic painful condition.

Ask them to tell you as much about their pain as possible. To do this, it is necessary to be fairly unstructured as you want them to talk 'openly' and give you plenty of information. However, questions might include:

- Tell me about your pain. Where is it? When did it start? How long has it lasted? How intense is it?

- What does the pain feel like? Note, for example, the words that patients use to describe their pain, such as ache, stabbing and shooting.

- What helps your pain? What makes it worse?

- How does the pain affect the quality of your life? Do you have difficulty sleeping? Does the pain wake you at night? Does it affect your mood and appetite?

- What could the nurses do to make your pain better or help you to cope with it?

- Do you take any medication for your pain? Do you have any side-effects from the medication? Do you use any coping strategies, for example relaxation?

- How do your family feel about your pain?

Each interview should take 20–30 minutes. Audiotaping it will save you having to take notes (but always ask the patient's permission first). Otherwise, write down as much as you can. Also include your observations of the patient (facial expression, body language and so on).

Time out   Reflect on the findings from your interview.

What are the implications for your practice?

From the information you have obtained, are there features that would be valuable for colleagues to know?

Does your clinical area have mechanisms in place for communicating some of your findings, such as a pain assessment tool in the care plan?

A study that explored the experiences of 75 people with chronic non-malignant pain found that pain adversely affected many dimensions of their lives (Seers and Friedli, 1996). The authors found that the most important factor for the patients was that their pain was believed; when you spoke with your patients about their chronic pain, they might have mentioned this to you. They may also have discussed the different activities they adopted to take their mind off the pain or help them to cope with it. Treatment may focus on trying to find a cause for the pain and treat this, but the underlying cause often cannot be treated, and patients are still left with their pain, feeling frustrated and disbelieved.

Care needs to reflect the social and cultural context of chronic pain and the impact that patients' backgrounds or social environments may have on how they respond to and cope with chronic pain. So many factors are known to influence how much distress pain will cause an individual. We all probably know of people who seem to cope with intolerable levels of pain with little if any obvious impact on the quality of their lives or the enjoyment of their social interaction. Other individuals, however, seem to become entirely consumed by pain; they constantly seek input from health care professionals in a desperate bid to have their pain explained. These unfortunate individuals will often have massive medical files as they are referred to doctor after doctor in an often fruitless attempt to find a 'cure'.

MANAGING CHRONIC PAIN

Before we consider some of the strategies that can be used, it is helpful to review how chronic pain is managed in your area. You will need to spend some time on this, the activities on the next page being suggested to enable you to explore this aspect more fully.

Think back to those patients who could be identified as experiencing chronic pain. Glance at some assessments and care plans – is their pain documented? The underdocumentation of pain is well reported (Albrecht et al., 1992), but documentation provides an important role in the management of pain as it allows us to share information and evaluate the effectiveness of interventions. Apart from a pain assessment tool, how else might you obtain information from patients about their pain?

Activity

List all the interventions that are used to manage chronic pain in your clinical practice, maybe bracketing them into pharmacological and non-pharmacological strategies.

Identify how each intervention relates to the Gate Control Theory of pain perception.

Do the interventions reflect the multidimensional nature of pain; that is, are both strategies incorporated into pain management, or are the pharmacological strategies the only ones made explicit?

All too often, health care professionals do not explore patients' views on their pain management, instead focusing on pharmacological interventions. Strategies such as relaxation, distraction, information giving, comfort (positioning) and skilled companionship (being with the patient) can all greatly contribute to the reduction of pain or help patients to 'cope' with their pain. Given that pain is multidimensional, it is logical that patients will benefit from a range of different approaches. The next section invites you to explore some of the pharmacological approaches to chronic pain and the use of pharmacological and non-pharmacological interventions.

Activity

Review the care plans relating to a problem of pain for three patients.

Are the problems clearly stated?

Are the goals realistic, measurable, achievable and patient centred?

Are the interventions all documented? Have the care plans been evaluated?

Write the results up in table format.

Reflect on your findings; what are your thoughts? You may be surprised to find how little is documented about the main symptom that first brought the patients into hospital or into contact with your clinical area.

PHARMACOLOGICAL APPROACHES TO PAIN MANAGEMENT

Drug therapy can be a very important part of treatment, and the reader is referred to Chapter 3 to review the main analgesics. In chronic (and acute) pain, adjuvant drug therapy is often used alongside other interventions. In chronic non-malignant pain, the treatment plan often encourages patients to reduce their consumption of analgesia and focus on coping strategies, reserving analgesic use for exacerbations. This is because this type of pain does not have an end-point – it is part of life, and people often need to learn how to live with their pain and minimise the discomfort. Having said that, there are, however, examples of chronic non-malignant pain that do respond to medication, and these will now be explored in more detail.

Adjuvant drug therapy

Adjuvant therapy describes drugs that do not have an obvious analgesic action but can, because of the complex origins of some types of pain, help to relieve pain in certain conditions and circumstances. In some cases, exactly how these drugs act is unknown. They can be given alongside traditional analgesia to improve pain relief, and the following will be considered in a little more detail:

- antidepressants
- anticonvulsants
- antispasmodic agents
- antihypertensives
- steroids
- benzodiazepines
- ketamine
- capsaicin
- bisphosphonates, chemotherapy and radiotherapy

Antidepressants

These drugs seem to provide analgesia by enhancing neurotransmitter activity at the terminals in the pain-modulating pathways. These are the pathways that originate in the brain and help the nervous system to tone down the incoming pain signals. Amitriptyline is one such drug often used to treat chronic pain. The dose given is usually much lower than that given to treat depression. When the drug is given to treat depression, the patient's response or improvement may take some time. When amitriptyline is given to enhance pain relief, however, some patients appear to respond quite quickly. Even though the doses are small, analgesia may also be enhanced because the patients may experience some antidepressant action or an improved quality of sleep, especially when the drug is given at night.

If the dose has to be increased in order to achieve a response, patients must be informed of the side-effects of these drugs, which may include sedation, constipation, a dry mouth and dizziness. At the low doses given for patients in pain, serious side-effects are rare. For further information see McQuay *et al.* (1996).

Activity

Think about how a patient might feel after visiting the GP for chronic pain and being prescribed an antidepressant.

What information would the patient also need to receive?

Many patients with chronic pain have pain without obvious evidence of the cause. This can be very demoralising as patients frequently undergo a battery of diagnostic tests that may be negative – but they still continue to have pain. When antidepressants are prescribed, the patient may feel that the doctor thinks it is 'all in my head' and does not really believe the pain. It is essential to explain that the antidepressant is thought to work on chemicals in the brain to reduce pain and is not being used to improve mood as the dose involved is very different. It is equally important to recognise that many people with chronic neuropathic pain will be depressed; successful management requires great sensitivity and understanding.

Anticonvulsants

These drugs provide analgesia for the shooting pains that occur with nerve damage. Like most of the drugs described here, their mechanism of action is not fully understood. It is thought that carbamazepine and phenytoin stabilise abnormal nerve firing as they do for patients experiencing convulsions. Carbamazepine has been found to be particularly useful for treating trigeminal neuralgia. Unfortunately, some patients suffer dizziness, epigastric pain, nausea and drowsiness. A new anticonvulsant, gabapentin, is showing promise for the treatment of some chronic neuropathic pain and appears to have fewer side-effects (Backonja et al., 1998; Rowbotham et al., 1998)

Antispasmodic agents

Baclofen is a substance used to treat smooth muscle spasm but can be quite effective in treating spasm caused by nerve damage, especially spasticity (Ochs et al., 1989; Penn et al., 1989). It is also thought to enhance the effect of one of the substances that the body produces to modulate pain. The principal side-effects are sedation, confusion and muscle weakness. Buscopan can be useful for relieving colic in acute postoperative pain but is often overlooked.

Antihypertensives

Clonidine is a very interesting drug that has been extensively studied. It is a central and peripheral alpha adrenergic blocker and can be an effective analgesic given spinally or via an epidural (Quan and Wandres, 1993). Clonidine can provide analgesia by modulating pain processing within the spinal cord and can be very effective when given epidurally for cancer pain, providing relief when all else has failed.

Steroids

These drugs are used quite frequently for the pain caused by a chronic inflammatory condition that has suddenly got worse. They are also used extensively when patients are suffering with advanced cancer pain. The drugs work in a variety of ways but probably provide analgesia by reducing the oedema that may be pressing on nerves or pain-sensitive structures. Their anti-inflammatory effects may also reduce the levels of the pain-producing chemicals found in damaged tissues. Steroids are not to be confused with non-steroidal anti-inflammatory

89

drugs (NSAIDs), which are analgesic drugs particularly useful for treating an acute pain, especially when there is an inflammatory response. NSAIDs are used in chronic pain management to treat an acute flare-up of a chronic inflammatory condition such as arthritis.

Benzodiazepines

These drugs, for example diazepam, are more commonly used to control acute musculoskeletal pain where there is muscle spasm and would rarely be appropriate for long-term use. Diazepam has been shown to bring pain relief for patients with a high level of anxiety or insomnia.

Ketamine

This is another very interesting drug in a class of its own. It is actually used in high doses as an intravenous general anaesthetic and in low doses has a strong analgesic action. It can, however, cause severe dysphoria (the opposite of euphoria) and terrible nightmares or dreams when used alone. Ketamine may be tried when a patient is not receiving relief from large doses of opioids, but its side-effects mean that it is reserved for 'difficult' cases. It is only available as a parenteral preparation and should therefore be given as a low-dose infusion, although some recent studies have been conducted using the parenteral preparation orally. The drug reduces activity at the NMDA (N-methyl-D-aspartate) receptor, thought to be one of the villains of pain control.

Capsaicin

This is a substance derived from chilli peppers and has been used for a variety of conditions in which pain has proved unresponsive to analgesia. Capsaicin is applied as a cream and is thought to deplete local sensory nerve terminals of substance P. Because capsaicin causes irritation of the skin, blind trials of its use have been difficult to carry out.

Bisphosphonates, chemotherapy and radiotherapy

These treatments are regularly used where pain is caused by a malignant tumour. Bisphosphonates can lessen pain in bones by reducing bone reabsorption. Chemotherapy and radiotherapy relieve pain by reducing tumour size, thereby alleviating pressure on local tissues, nerves or organs.

The role of opioids in the management of non-malignant pain

Before we leave this section, opioids must be considered. Their use in non-malignant pain has been highly controversial, some clinicians believing them to be wholly inappropriate. This view is now changing a little as people with cancer now 'live with cancer', and many are prescribed opioids over months or even years. Glynn *et al.* (1991) offer the following guidelines for the use of opioids in non-malignant pain. They should only be used when:

- all other treatments have failed
- it is evident that the opioids do relieve the pain
- the patient, supported by his or her family/carers is willing to use opioids
- other doctors involved in the patient's care are willing for them to be used
- appropriate follow-up care is planned.

REGIONAL NERVE BLOCKS

In addition to the previous pharmacological interventions, there are a range of special procedures that can be performed by a trained physician to interrupt the nerve pathways. It is not appropriate to consider these here; further information can be found in King and Jacob (1993). It is important not to neglect the role of the nurse during these procedures, nurses' prime responsibility usually being to provide safety, comfort, reassurance and information.

NON-PHARMACOLOGICAL STRATEGIES FOR MANAGING CHRONIC PAIN

The effective management of chronic pain has to incorporate a range of strategies that have a physical and a psychosocial basis. The following non-pharmacological strategies can be extremely helpful in reducing the perception of pain and helping the person to live and cope with his or her pain. It is important to discuss the goal of pain treatment with the person concerned. For example, with chronic pain caused by arthritis, it might be unrealistic to have 'no pain' as a goal, but the person may wish to have a pain level that still allows them to take the children to school.

Pain is a multidimensional phenomenon involving sensory, emotional, motivational, environmental and cognitive components. The following sections reflect the diverse and useful range of strategies available to reduce the impact of pain on a person's life, the intention being to widen approaches to managing pain and to provide you with an opportunity to understand how you might contribute. At this point, however, it must be stressed that nurses should only provide therapies for which they have been appropriately trained, abiding by the UKCC Code of Conduct. Some therapies, such as heat and cold therapy, require basic knowledge. Other strategies, although many still lack regulation, can be practised following the completion of one of the vast range of courses currently available. These courses range from 1–2 study days in simple massage to a degree course in osteopathy.

PHYSICAL TECHNIQUES FOR MANAGING PAIN

We are now entering the realms of complementary approaches to pain management. In the past, some of these interventions have been slow to gain clinical acceptability because of a lack of rigorous research, but this is now changing (Stevenson, 1995). Some cognitive and behavioural therapies have been tested scientifically and have shown clear beneficial effects, but for the most part it appears that much of the existing research is inconclusive because of common methodological problems with the primary studies (Carroll, 1997).

In practice, many people derive great benefit, which is not always measurable, from complementary approaches this being particularly relevant for people suffering pain. Relief from pain may not always be the patient's goal: well-being and improved sleep may be other important outcomes. These therapies should not be underestimated as they will often provide some relief when drugs and other treatments fail. As we are now in a climate of evidence-based practice and clinical governance, there is a need not only to be aware of current research, but also to conduct large randomised controlled trials, however difficult these may be in practice.

Acupuncture

Acupuncture has been practised for thousands of years. Although still not fully understood, it is certainly gaining credibility in Western medicine as a valid treatment for certain types of pain. The technique involves placing fine solid needles into the skin at acupoints along energy pathways termed meridians, which are described in classical Chinese medicine.

More than a decade of research has provided scientists with a reasonable explanation of how acupuncture works. There is evidence that acupuncture needles stimulate sensory nerves in the skin and muscles, and that these signal to the spinal cord and midbrain. This type of stimulation results in pain modulation, probably via the release of the body's own opioids – endorphins. It is also thought that the use of acupuncture may cause the pituitary to discharge pain-blocking chemicals and anti-inflammatory agents into the circulation.

Acupuncture should always be conducted by those trained in its art as a range of adverse effects, such as pneumothorax and infection, have been associated with its use. It is a therapy that can be valuable for many conditions other than pain relief (Mann, 1999). There are certainly patients who have derived considerable benefit from acupuncture, but it is often tried as a last resort when all other treatments have either caused more problems or failed to provide any relief.

Acupressure

This therapy is reputed to be even older than acupuncture, although it is not as widely practised. Acupressure is said to produce much the same effect as acupuncture but does not involve needles. Finger or hand pressure is used over the acupoints, which feature along the same energy pathways that form the basis of acupuncture. One form of acupressure is the use of 'sea bands', elasticated bands, usually

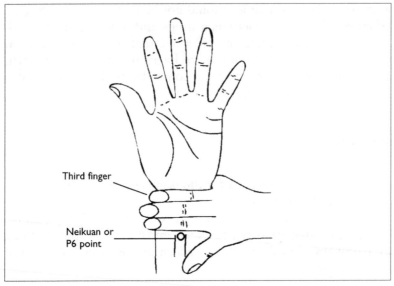

Third finger

Neikuan or
P6 point

Figure 4.1   Acupuncture/acupressure point of nausea/PONV

about 3 cm wide, which have a small, hard button attached to the inside. They can be worn on the wrist with the button positioned over the P6 point (Figure 4.1). Although traditionally used to treat sea-sickness, several researchers have in the past reported the benefits of using them to treat postoperative nausea and vomiting (Bill and Dundee, 1988; Barsoum *et al.*, 1990; Phillips and Leicester, 1993).

Massage

Massage has certainly been very useful in acute pain and would, there-fore, probably be beneficial for chronic pain sufferers. It is thought to provide pain relief in a variety of ways. The stimulation of the skin may increase the circulation, which contributes to reducing swelling and promoting healing. Touch and massage can stimulate the large diameter A beta fibres which close the gate. The personal attention and relaxation associated with massage can generate a feeling of well-being and modify pain perception. Many sports people who sustain a painful injury find that their muscles and any damaged tissue respond quickly to moderately deep massage, and they are able to return to the sports field more rapidly. Babies especially have been seen to obtain relief from the pain of colic using gentle massage. When pain is chronic, research has also shown the benefits of massage for patients with arthritis and fibromyalgia syndromes.

Aromatherapy

Aromatherapy involves the use of essential oils distilled from plants. In addition to having wonderful fragrances, they are also claimed to have specific therapeutic properties that work on the limbic system to reduce tension and stress. They can be used to promote sleep (lavender) and relieve pain. Certain oils, such as tea tree oil, are known to possess an antibacterial action. The oils can be administered in a number of ways: massaged into the skin, dropped neat onto a handkerchief or pillow, used as room sprays, evaporated in special burners, placed in compresses or added to bath water.

Reflexology

This therapy, like acupuncture, represents a revival of an ancient practice. The therapy is based on the idea that every part of the body has a reflex point on the foot and hand. Therapists use their fingers and hands to produce simple, safe pressure. When an area of tenderness is found, the therapist concentrates on that area by pressure in a specific manner to either stimulate or sedate the reflex. It is claimed that the therapy can bring pain relief by 'normalising' organ function and can be particularly useful for dysmenorrhoea, constipation, irritable bowel syndrome, urinary retention and premenstrual symptoms.

Transcutaneous electrical nerve stimulation

Transcutaneous electrical nerve stimulator devices were briefly described in Chapter 3; they are thought to work by sending a weak electrical current through the skin to stimulate the sensory nerve endings. This feels like a prickly, buzzing sensation but should not be unpleasant. It is also thought that transcutaneous electrical nerve stimulation (TENS) may help to close the 'gate' in the thalamus of the brain, where pain nerve endings and ordinary touch sensation converge before their final distribution to the cortex of the brain. Some research also suggests that TENS may stimulate the release of extra pain-relieving chemicals within the brain and spinal cord. TENS can work for all sorts of pain but is usually helpful in relieving rheumatic-type aching in joints and muscles, low back pain, amputation stump pain and neuralgia. For further reading on TENS, see Walsh (1997).

Many companies lease TENS machines, along with simple instructions (for example, for labour pain and the muscle and joint pain associated with arthritis), to patients, or they can often be purchased in health shops. They are popular because they have no side-effects, and many patients derive considerable relief from their pain. Nurses need to know how they work so that they can teach their patients to use the machines safely and confidently.

The research on the effectiveness of TENS for postoperative pain has been inconclusive. Where patients do derive benefit from the system it would seem prudent to continue using it.

Activity

Find out where you might obtain a TENS machine in your hospital and/or community.

Identify what you would need to learn in order to recommend its use to a patient or friend and teach them how to use it.

Speak to someone who has used a machine and find out how they use it for pain relief – try it yourself too! In many hospitals, physiotherapists are a good source of expertise.

Heat therapy

We all know how good soaking in a warm bath can be: heating the tissues of the body can be very comforting. Warmth to the skin may be another way of closing the gate mechanism in the spinal cord. The conscious feeling of warmth tends to suppress the awareness of pain and helps to promote mental and physical relaxation.

Raising the temperature of damaged tissue may speed up the metabolic process, improve circulation by vasodilatation, reduce oedema and accelerate repair. The heat of a warm bath before activity can reduce the viscosity of synovial fluid, which can reduce painful stiffness in joints with diseases such as arthritis. Starting the day with a warm bath may enable sufferers to function more comfortably. Heat is a useful therapy for backache, rheumatic conditions and pain arising from scar tissue or adhesions. Interestingly, when heat is used to treat stomach ache, it can reduce acidity within 5 minutes. Heat should, however, never be used immediately following tissue damage as it will increase swelling.

Cold therapy

Cold therapy may also be a way of stimulating nerves to bring about pain modulation, although its value in chronic pain is limited. With a burn injury, however, plunging the area into cold water will halt the actual tissue damage as well as temporarily ease the pain. In fact, if the water is cold enough, the patient will cease to feel the pain from the burn at all. Cold can be applied to treat pain in the form of wrapped crushed ice, and gel-filled cold packs that are stored in the fridge are commercially available. Even a bag of frozen peas can make all the difference following an acute bruising injury. In some acute conditions, cold causes vasoconstriction, which reduces the inflammatory response and can limit further damage. It is essential to wrap any bagged ice in a towel or cotton to protect the skin from an ice burn.

PSYCHOLOGICAL INTERVENTIONS

Previous experience, current mood, alertness and expectations all play a part in our response to pain. Whether we feel we have control over an event is an important determinant of how we respond (Walker *et al.*, 1989). We can use our brain to influence our experience of pain. Psychological techniques include biofeedback, hypnosis and cognitive strategies (see Williams, 1997). This section will consider some of the strategies that are easy to use and helpful.

Relaxation

Strategies can utilise a range of interventions. Progressive relaxation is easy to learn and effective. Usually starting at the feet and working up, muscle groups are selected and purposefully tensed for several seconds before being relaxed. Anxiety and muscle relaxation produce opposite physiological states and therefore cannot exist together.

Seers (1997) describes the impact of a community-based programme using relaxation skills for sufferers of chronic non-malignant pain. The findings revealed that those patients taught relaxation skills experienced a decrease in their pain intensity and an improvement in sleep in both the short and the longer term. It is well worth reading Seer's excellent paper as it considers the wider issues concerning the provision of pain services for those people experiencing chronic non-malignant pain.

Activity

Get into a comfortable position and bring your shoulders up towards your ears. Hold the position for 10 seconds. Then slowly let your shoulders down as low as you possibly can – keep going!

What do you notice about your shoulders now?

Were you aware of the muscle tensions before you did this exercise?

Guided imagery

Guided imagery involves a mental picture of reality or fantasy and usually involves all five senses. It is a technique that is relatively easy to use and can be helpful for chronic pain and short painful procedures. Like other non-pharmacological strategies, it should not take the place of analgesia but complement it. Try to make sure that there will be no interruptions and that the environment is warm. Choosing a subject to explore, through the senses, should be agreed between the patient and nurse – maybe a holiday or an activity the patient enjoys.

The following 'time out' is an example of guided imagery. Imagining the scene, see whether you can visualise the image so clearly that you can take your mind off what is going on around you. Imagery that involves natural experiences – the warmth of the sun or sparkling light on the sea – is good to include. You have to concentrate quite hard, some people finding this easier than others.

Time out It is a warm summer evening and the wind gently rustles through the leaves on the trees. You are sitting beneath an oak tree and can feel the slightly damp grass beneath you and the warm rays of sun on your skin. In the distance, you hear the sounds of laughter from children playing and the splash of water as they paddle and jump. The fragrant smell of freshly cut grass and heady scent of roses mingle together...

Music therapy

This can work as an excellent cognitive therapy, with the added benefit that some pieces of music will soothe and relax the listener. Music has been shown to cause the release of the body's own opioids, endorphins, as well as acting as a cue for relaxation therapy.

A detailed review of studies on the effects of relaxation and music on postoperative pain concluded that they reduced the pain, especially the affective (emotional) component (Good, 1996). A personal stereo can be used to listen to music, the volume being increased or decreased in response to the pain; it can even be used at work or while being active. The fear of the pain occurring at work can sometimes be particularly worrying so interventions that are discreet and easily utilised are important.

All the above strategies centre around involvement with treatment and exercising a personal sense of control. How individuals perceive their control over a situation will influence how they deal with and respond to it. People with an external locus of control style appear to experience more intense pain than those with an internal locus of control style (Bates *et al.*, 1993). For example, feelings of helplessness are a predictor of higher levels of pain in patients with phantom limb pain (Hill *et al.*, 1995). In chronic pain, treatments that encourage an internal locus of control, such as the self-treatment strategies mentioned above, would appear to have the greatest long-term benefit compared with treatments that are just 'done to' patients.

TRUSTING THERAPEUTIC RELATIONSHIPS

Creating a trusting nurse–patient relationship is often ignored as a therapeutic intervention. The nursing partnership has been viewed as a way of looking at what happens when the nurse offers expertise to a person who is experiencing a health-related problem (Christensen, 1993). This partnership can be an essential component in the management of pain. The ability to convey trust and empathy is a skilled nursing action that requires a partnership in care in which patients and their families are central. Someone experiencing pain is especially vulnerable, and the nurse can be instrumental in helping them cope with the pain.

Time out　Reflect on the notes you made earlier in this chapter following your interviews with people experiencing chronic pain.
Did you notice anything about the 'effect' of taking time to talk with them about their pain?
What do you think you were conveying to the patients when you chatted with them, and how might this influence their pain experience?

Living with pain day and night, and feeling isolated, depressed and frightened, is devastating. This may be compounded if no physical cause can be found for the pain and an endless round of hospital appointments have left the sufferer feeling that no one believes him. Having others believe the pain has been found to be crucial for non-malignant chronic pain sufferers (Seers and Friedli, 1996). By discussing pain with your patient, it is likely that you conveyed belief in their pain as well as trust and empathy. This activity of talking openly about pain can ultimately prove highly beneficial in helping patients to cope with what may prove to be an incurable condition.

SOCIAL ACTIVITIES

With chronic non-malignant pain, sufferers often become isolated and depressed as a result of the relentless pain they experience. The vicious circle only causes them to withdraw further, and they often no longer participate in the social activities they once enjoyed so much. Facilitating them to engage in social interaction is important. Meeting friends will help to take their mind off the pain as well as increasing their self-esteem. When pharmacological strategies and medical intervention fail to bring any relief, supporting patients to return to as normal a lifestyle as possible is sometimes the most realistic goal.

Over a period of time, certain patients with pain of unknown aetiology will go on to develop pain behaviours and negative coping strategies, and will adopt the 'sick role'. This results in their withdrawing further from their environment; it alters their role in society so that they become less active, participate less and become totally centred on their own pain. Their management can become very challenging indeed. The final chapter of this book will cover further some of the issues surrounding the care for patients who fall into this category.

EXERCISE

For patients suffering chronic benign pain, establishing a programme of structured physical exercise should be incorporated into strategies to control pain. Although these might at first prove difficult, exercise is thought to be beneficial for the following reasons:

- it increases mobility
- it enables social interaction
- it decreases muscle strain and reduces muscle spasm
- it stimulates natural endorphins
- it produces stimuli that compete with pain, thereby reducing the perception of pain
- it reduces fatigue by increasing stamina
- it maintains cardiovascular fitness
- it reduces bone demineralisation.

Time out   Reflect back on your conversations.
Did your patients talk about their social life at all?
Did they still participate in social events or visits to friends?
If they had stopped, why was this?
How could they start some of these again?

PROFESSIONAL COLLABORATION IN PAIN MANAGEMENT

A variety of professionals can make an important contribution to providing effective pain relief, both as individuals and as part of a specialist team. In the previous section, a range of interventions were identified for the management of pain; in some cases, for example TENS, physiotherapists or specialist nurses may be consulted for their expertise and contribution.

Activity

Consider the health care professionals in your clinical area who have a role in the management of chronic pain. Make short notes on each of their roles. Now interview each on how they perceive their role in the management of chronic pain.

Are there any other health care professionals in your hospital or community who have an interest in pain?

How do you access their input?

How could you improve collaboration between the many professions with an interest or role in pain management?

It can be quite surprising to discover how many different health care professionals have an input to or interest in pain management. All may have their own expertise and approach. When this is communicated effectively and these professionals work together, the impact can be immense. The following sections consider how multiprofessional teamwork has made a difference in chronic pain.

CHRONIC PAIN CLINICS

The concept of the chronic pain clinic was initially proposed by two enthusiastic anaesthetists, John Lloyd and Samuel Lipton, in the 1960s. The techniques originally used were nerve blocks and pharmacological intervention, but clinics now utilise a range of strategies from acupuncture and exercise to biofeedback and psychotherapy, involving a range of professionals. These multidisciplinary pain clinics have become increasingly popular and have adopted a variety of formats. Patients may be referred to a chronic pain clinic by their general practitioner or a consultant who has been managing their care. The clinics vary greatly in their structure and management.

An outcome study of a multidisciplinary chronic pain programme found a significant increase in physical functioning, 48 per cent of the treatment group returning to work compared with none of the non-treated group (Deardorff *et al.*, 1991). An inpatient programme of 1 month's duration is described by Crabbe (1989), but others can be accessed on a daily basis. See O'Hara (1996) for more detail on the structure of such teams and the role of individual professionals.

The provision of chronic pain services in the UK is increasingly being scrutinised as the current format of expensive services for a minority of people makes neither moral nor fiscal sense. Seers (1997) emphasises this point in the rationale to provide a community-based service for people suffering with chronic non-malignant pain using a very simple and cheap intervention (relaxation training). Nurses are ideally placed to develop such services to meet the needs of patients.

Activity

Find out where your nearest chronic pain clinic is situated and identify how patients are referred to it.

What facilities does it offer, and how does it evaluate the success of its programmes?

Write this up on a couple of sides of A4 paper.

As previously mentioned, you might discover that such services are few and far between and that interventions might instead focus on pharmacological agents. Is there a role here for the nurse to develop services utilising some of the non-pharmacological interventions previously discussed in this chapter? A nurse may already be involved in the clinic, but in what capacity? Does the role of the nurse actively contribute to helping the patient? Many questions can be asked, but the future looks promising, with a wider recognition of chronic pain.

The need to provide care that reaches more people, helping them to improve the quality of their lives, could become a higher priority in the years to come.

McQuay et al. (1997) have reviewed evidence on the effective treatments for chronic pain, focusing on individual treatments rather than the provision of pain clinics. They describe in detail how the reviews were evaluated. Their findings can be summarised thus:

- *TENS* – Evidence suggests it to be beneficial when used in large doses, its effectiveness increasing over time. More research is needed.
- *Relaxation* – There is a lack of evidence for its effectiveness.
- *Regional blocks* – Using guanethidine has no positive effect on chronic pain.
- *Epidural corticosteroids* – These are effective in the short term.
- *Injecting corticosteroids to shoulder joints* – This treatment is not effective.
- *Minor analgesics* – These are important in chronic pain. Codeine (NNT = 17) is a poor choice, but ibuprofen (NNT = 2.5) is better.
- *Centrally acting drugs* – These comprise an effective treatment (NNT about 2.5).
- *Topical NSAIDs* – Topical NSAIDs are effective for rheumatological conditions (NNT = 3).
- *Psychological interventions* such as cognitive behaviour therapies – Thirty five trials of such interventions in pain therapy have shown a large and sustainable improvement in targeted outcomes.
- *Cost* – There is evidence to suggest that pain clinics reduce health care costs by £1000 per patient per year. Pain clinics generate savings equal to twice their running cost.

The NNT, or number needed to treat, is the efficacy index of an analgesia; an NNT of 2–4 indicating effective treatment.

CONCLUSION

When pain does not have a foreseeable end and may have to be endured throughout life, the nurse can help the person and his or her family to come to terms with this situation and cope with the pain. Educating patients and their families about pain, and drawing on their coping skills, gives the person some control over their life.

This chapter has focused on collecting data from clinical practice to help you to explore how chronic pain is currently being managed in your area. It has given you a framework against which your own experiences and environment can be compared. It is anticipated that this will provide you with the enthusiasm and knowledge to analyse the current management of chronic pain in your practice area and identify methods of influencing change.

After a break, try the multiple-choice questionnaire below in order to self-assess your understanding so far.

Suggested further reading

Bowman, J. (1994) Experiencing the chronic pain phenomenon: a study. *Rehabilitation Nursing*, 19(2): 91–5.

Gadsby, G. and Flowerdew, M. (1997) Nerve stimulation for low back pain. *Nursing Standard*, 11(43): 32–7.

Haythornthwaite, J.A., Menefee, L.A., Heinberg, L.J. and Clarke, M.R. (1998) Pain coping strategies predict perceived control over pain. *Pain*, **77**: 33–9.

McCaffery, M. and Beebe, A. (1994) *Pain: Clinical Manual for Nursing Practice*, London, C.V. Mosby, Non-invasive Pain Relief Measures (Chapter 6) and Chronic Non-malignant Pain: Special Considerations (Chapter 7).

Price, S. and Price, L. (1995) *Aromatherapy for Health Professionals*, Edinburgh, Churchill Livingstone.

Richardson, A. (1997) Cancer pain and its management. In Thomas, V.N. (ed.) *Pain: Its Nature and Management*, London, Baillière Tindall, pp. 194–219.

Seers, K. and Friedli, B. (1996) The patients' experiences of their chronic non-malignant pain. *Journal of Advanced Nursing*, **24**: 1160–8.

Sindhu, F. (1996) Are non-pharmacological nursing interventions for the management of pain effective: a meta analysis. *Journal of Advanced Nursing*, **24**: 1152–9.

Managing Chronic Pain

MULTIPLE-CHOICE QUESTIONNAIRE

1. Why is it important to differentiate between chronic malignant and chronic non-malignant pain?

    a. Chronic non-malignant pain has a foreseeable end ☐
    b. Analgesia is the only intervention for chronic malignant pain ☐
    c. The approach to using analgesics is different for the two types of pain ☐
    d. Chronic non-malignant pain responds well to analgesia ☐

2. Why should the assessment and management of pain be documented?

    a. It allows the effectiveness of interventions to be evaluated ☐
    b. It is good practice and professional ☐
    c. It allows other professionals to see how pain is being managed ☐
    d. Documentation formalises the management of pain ☐

3. 'Adjuvant therapy' is the term given to which of the following?

    a. Drugs used to treat the side-effects of analgesia ☐
    b. Drugs used to complement analgesics ☐
    c. Drugs used to reverse analgesics ☐
    d. Drugs used to treat anxiety and depression ☐

4. Which drug(s) is frequently used as a treatment for chronic pain experienced by patients with or without any obvious pathology?

    a. Steroids ☐
    b. Ketamine ☐
    c. Bisphosphonates ☐
    d. Antidepressants ☐

5. How is it suggested that acupuncture works for the management of pain?

    a. By stimulating the meridians ☐
    b. By stimulating motor nerves in the skin ☐
    c. By taking a person's mind off the pain experience ☐
    d. By stimulating the sensory nerves in the skin, which causes the body to release endorphins ☐

6. Which nerve fibres are beneficially stimulated when using TENS?

    a. C fibres ☐
    b. A beta fibres ☐
    c. Motor nerve fibres ☐
    d. A delta fibres ☐

MULTIPLE-CHOICE QUESTIONNAIRE (cont'd)

7. Which of the following has been shown to have a specific effect on gastric acidity?

   a. TENS ☐

   b. Aromatherapy ☐

   c. Acupressure ☐

   d. Heat therapy ☐

8. Which factor has been shown to be the most important for chronic non-malignant pain sufferers?

   a. Having others believe their pain ☐

   b. Regular consultations with doctors ☐

   c. Rest and the avoidance of physical activity ☐

   d. Regular analgesia ☐

9. Who set up the concept of the chronic pain clinic?

   a. Melzack and Wall ☐

   b. Dame Cicely Saunders ☐

   c. Arthur Lipman ☐

   d. John Lloyd and Samuel Lipton ☐

10. If you were to identify an improvement that could be made in the management of chronic pain in your area, which would be the most important activity for you to undertake first?

   a Collect information to identify current practices ☐

   b. Talk with patients and relatives ☐

   c. Read the current literature on the subject and so on ☐

   d. Implement the 'improvement' ☐

ANSWERS FOR THE MULTIPLE-CHOICE QUESTIONNAIRE

1 . **c. The approach to using analgesics is different for the two types of pain**; the use of analgesia in chronic malignant pain is an important intervention for ensuring that the pain is kept within tolerable limits. The fear of tolerance or addiction is not an issue, and the analgesia should be given in sufficient doses and at sufficient intervals to ensure effective pain relief. In chronic non-malignant pain, patients take responsibility for their pain and should not rely solely on analgesia; analgesics are often ineffective and elicit unwanted side-effects.

2. **a. It allows the effectiveness of interventions to be evaluated**; the documentation of pain assessment and management allows us to share the

effectiveness of the selected interventions. Without this record, the patient's response to these interventions cannot be evaluated. This renders interventions *ad hoc*, resulting in pain management that is often ineffective. It should be noted that all the other answers were also important, although less so.

3. **b. Drugs used to complement analgesics**; although not necessarily analgesics in themselves, many of the adjuvant therapies will result in enhanced analgesia when used with traditional analgesic drugs, or on their own to treat specific conditions.

4. **d. Antidepressants**; particularly amitriptyline. Steroids are used for inflammatory conditions. Ketamine is an anaesthetic induction agent that is an NMDA receptor antagonist, NMDA being thought to be responsible for the 'wind-up' phenomenon of pain. Bisphosphonates are used to treat the pain arising from bone reabsorbtion that occurs with certain tumours.

5. **d. By stimulating the sensory nerves in the skin, which causes the body to release endorphins**; the acupuncture needles stimulate the sensory nerves in the skin. These send impulses to the brain via the spinal cord and midbrain, causing a modulation response. As a result, the body is stimulated to release its own analgesics – endorphins.

6. **b. A beta fibres**, the touch and vibration sensation fibres. They conduct the impulses faster than other nerve fibres, and it is thought that the activity generated by this inhibits the activity of the pain fibres within the spinal cord.

7. **d. Heat therapy**; heat therapy has been shown to reduce gastric acidity within 5 minutes. There are no data to support a similar response following aromatherapy, acupressure or TENS.

8. **a. Having others believe their pain** has been shown to be the most important factor (Seers and Friedli, 1996). Patients may feel that other people do not believe their pain, especially if a cause cannot be found. All the remaining answers have been shown to impact negatively on the pain experience for chronic non-malignant pain suffers.

9. **d. John Lloyd and Samuel Lipton.**

10. **a. Collect information to identify current practices**; this baseline information will be invaluable in establishing what is currently happening so that when you have introduced your 'improvement' (for example, a relaxation strategy), you will be able to collect more data and establish whether the improvement in fact made a difference in practice. The process of collecting information will facilitate getting your colleagues involved in being part of the change. Answers b and c described activities in which you could engage when collecting the information. Making a change without a, b or c is a recipe for failure!

5

Recognising the barriers to effective pain relief

LEARNING OUTCOMES

On completion of this chapter, the student will be able to:

■ Critically discuss the effects of the inappropriate knowledge and attitudes of health care professionals on the effective management of pain

■ Identify factors that contribute to patients' minimising their pain, and strategies that might reduce their impact

■ Evaluate current practices that might contribute to ineffective pain management

INDICATIVE READING

Brockopp, D.Y., Brockopp, G., Warden, S., Wilson, J., Carpenter, J.S. and Vandeveer, B. (1998) Barrier to change: a pain management project. *International Journal of Nursing Studies*, **35**: 226–32.

Carr, E.C.J. (1997) Overcoming barriers to effective pain control. *Professional Nurse*, **12**(6): 412–16.

Mackintosh, C. (1994) Do nurses provide adequate postoperative pain relief? *British Journal of Nursing*, **3**(7): 342–7.

Niven, C. (1994) *Coping with Labour Pain: The Midwife's Role*. London, Chapman & Hall. (for midwifery students.)

Watt-Watson, J. (1987) Nurses' knowledge of pain issues: a survey. *Journal of Pain and Symptom Management*, **2**(4): 207–11.

BACKGROUND

Pain control is a contemporary issue that is of immense importance because of the devastating and dehumanising effects that it can have upon an individual indiscriminately crossing age groups and client groups. The focus of this chapter is primarily on the health care professional, the patient, organisations and their roles in pain management. The management of pain in vulnerable and challenging patient groups may create unique demands, which are discussed in more detail in Chapters 6 and 7.

Nursing the patient who is experiencing pain requires contemporary knowledge, skilled interventions (both pharmacological and non-pharmacological) and attitudes that convey trust, empathy and an honest belief in the patient. This may seem simple, yet the real world presents daily complexities and challenges confronting clinicians managing pain. This chapter draws on well-documented 'barriers' to effective pain management and outlines appropriate strategies in an attempt to lessen their impact. In reflecting on your own clinical practice and a sense of having 'been there', recognising the barriers can be frustrating. However, we hope that this chapter will enthuse, motivate and invite you to feel more confident in contributing to effective pain management.

HEALTH CARE PROFESSIONALS

Griepp (1992) reviewed 15 pain studies and identified the 'knowledge deficit' of professionals as being the most prevalent causative factor of inadequate pain management. Although effective analgesic techniques are available, they are frequently not used. The reasons for this have been attributed to physicians' failure to prescribe effective analgesia and their adherence to dosage schedules known to be ineffective, as well as to the inappropriate attitudes and beliefs of both nurses and doctors (McCaffery et al., 1990; Clarke et al., 1996).

Nurses are not the only ones who have been found to have a deficiency in their pain knowledge. A survey of 27 medical schools revealed that four undertook no formal teaching on pain control, the remainder averaged only 3.5 hours during a 5-year course (Marcer and Deighton, 1988). It is worrying that this important work is now several years old yet no replication of the study has been undertaken. Wallace et al. (1997) lament that few studies have been conducted to evaluate the effects of pain education on practice, as most studies have focused on pain assessment or documentation. The provision of continuing professional education in pain management is not well reported, but it was recently suggested as a topic by the General Medical Council (1997). Overall, it would appear that the attention to this important area has been greatly neglected and the educational preparation of professionals remains inadequate.

Activity

Find three research articles on 'pain and education'.

What were the researchers trying to find out?

What methods did they use to answer the research question(s)?

Most researchers are trying to assess the knowledge and attitudes of health care professionals. The usual method for doing this is a questionnaire. Questionnaires can be helpful to measure how much people know about a subject, but it does not tell you whether they use this knowledge in their practice. Someone filling in the questionnaire may give all the right answers but not have the confidence to use the knowledge in practice. Research using other methods such as observation and measuring patient outcomes might give a more insightful answer. It would be logical to expect that practitioners with a high level of pain knowledge would give better care (as patients experienced less pain) than practitioners with less knowledge. A recent literature review of nurse education highlighted the inadequacies of evaluation for those educational programmes provided (Franke *et al.*, 1996).

The following are examples of some of the common misconceptions surrounding pain that are held by practitioners and reported in research studies:

- Patients should expect pain in hospital.
- Obvious pathology, abnormal test results and the type of surgery determine the existence and intensity of pain.
- Patients in pain always have observable signs.
- Chronic pain is not as serious as acute pain.
- Patients will always tell you when they have pain.
- One type of pain intervention, for example analgesia, is sufficient to relieve pain.
- Addiction and respiratory depression are major problems with opioid use.

III

- Patients should have pain before being given analgesia.
- Patients who laugh and chat to visitors cannot have that much pain.

Time out   Think about pain management in your clinical area.

Do any of the above statements ring true?

Why do you think these views are held?

The effective management of pain relies on the teamwork of different professionals, each with a valuable contribution. As already mentioned, it is essential that they have the appropriate knowledge to manage pain effectively. Even more important is the ability to work together and communicate effectively, yet conflict and misunderstanding can make working as a team difficult (Brockopp *et al.*, 1998).

Activity

Think of a patient you have cared for who has experienced pain.

Reflect on the role of the different professionals involved in that person's care.

Was there any difficulty or conflict between the professionals, or between the patient and a professional?

Communication between professionals is sometimes not always as clear as it could be. A nurse might identify a patient who is experiencing a lot of pain and ask the doctor to change the analgesic prescription. The doctor might find that the patient does not appear to have much pain and think that the analgesia prescription is adequate. Conflict occurs when the nurse bathes the patient and finds that turning him causes pain and distress. If the doctor and nurse had discussed this person's pain together (with the patient), this might not have happened.

IMPROVING PRACTICE

case history

Pilkington Ward is a busy adult oncology ward. A recent pain audit revealed that some patients experienced unrelieved pain. When the ward staff received the feedback from the audit, they were rather dismayed as they thought that they had been quite good with pain control. One nurse said 'well, we do our best, but the problem is that the patients refuse analgesia when it is offered'. Using a problem-solving approach, the ward team decided to conduct a small improvement project on 'patients refusing analgesia'.

1. Identifying the problem – how many patients refuse analgesia and why?
A sheet of paper was taped to the inside of the drug trolley, nurses noting down when patients were asked whether they would like analgesia and what their response was (acceptance or refusal). If patients refused analgesia, they were asked why.

● Seventy per cent of all patients asked whether they would like an analgesic refused.

  Reasons: Most patients preferred not to take analgesia, would wait until later or did not have pain.

2. Making some small changes
Many patients did not see that good pain relief was important or preferred to tolerate the pain rather than endure the unpleasant side-effects of analgesia (such as constipation). It also became apparent that not all nurses asked patients about their pain in the same way, and that there was a lack of pain assessment. The team got together and decided to make three small changes in an attempt to encourage patients to accept analgesia when offered:

● On each drug round, the nurse would ask patients to score their pain on a 0–10 scale, which would then be noted on the TPR chart. This would enable nurses to evaluate the effectiveness of previous analgesia and encourage patients to accept analgesia based on their previous pain score.

● A patient information sheet on analgesia was designed. This included why it was important to be comfortable to move, how to manage side-effects and what to do if pain relief was not effective. This sheet was given to all patients at the preadmission clinic and on admission to the ward.

● To meet the education needs of the nurses on the ward, a 'tip of the week' was created, which could be a couple of sentences about the key findings from a piece of research, with the reference. This was laminated and taped to the inside of the drug trolley.

3. Evaluating the effectiveness
After 6 months, a re-audit revealed that only 58 per cent of patients now refused analgesia. This was positive feedback and encouraged the nurses to look at other ways in which they might continue to reduce the number of patients refusing analgesia.

Activity

Design a short questionnaire to give to your own professional group. Ideally, this should take only a few minutes (no more than 10) to complete.

Ask a few questions about their knowledge of and attitudes towards pain.

See below for an example.

For example:

- How would you define pain?
- What is the chance of someone becoming addicted to morphine if they receive regular opioids, for trauma, over a 2-week period?

  a. 30 per cent
  b. less than 1 per cent
  c. 60 per cent
  d. Don't know

When you have collected this information, try to summarise your findings; putting the answers into a table format can help. Then write one side of A4 (or more if you wish) on your findings and the implications of your survey in relation to the management of patients' pain. Reflect on the process of this activity. How did you feel about carrying out the survey and the information you found?

Alternatively, try the following. You may be able to obtain from your local hospital or university library a video and booklet called *Partnering Patients to Manage Pain after Surgery* (Carr and Mann, 1998). The video uses the patient's perspective to consider how nursing can actively contribute to reducing pain. Through this combined medium, evidence is explored that challenges past misconceptions and contemporary barriers to effective pain management. Try watching this in a small group before discussing the findings. Could you apply any of the suggestions to your clinical area?

Obtaining information from your own practice area, or seeing what is happening elsewhere, can be very interesting. It may act as a catalyst for conversations between colleagues and for suggestions on improving practice. It can also raise the 'awareness' of a particular problem or issue. If the findings are not very good or give rise for concern, there may be feelings of guilt or anxiety to do something.

Activity

Now go back and read some of those articles on health care professionals' knowledge and attitudes in relation to pain.

Compare your findings with those written in the literature. What do you find?

You will have found, through your own reading, that a lack of knowledge and the inappropriate attitudes of health care professionals are two of the major causes of the ineffective management of patients' pain. Some of the very early research in the 1970s suggested this (Marks and Sachar, 1973), yet inadequate knowledge and inappropriate attitudes continue to be a significant problem. Did your findings bear any similarity to those of other research in the area, for example the findings of Closs (1996)?

PATIENT BARRIERS TO EFFECTIVE PAIN MANAGEMENT

Effective pain management can be challenging when patients are unable or have difficulty in communicating their pain, for example with children, neonates, people with learning disabilities and those whose culture is different from that of the health care professional. These issues are given greater consideration in Chapter 6. The following sections consider some of the everyday reasons why patients may minimise their pain. Despite the best will in the world, there are times when patients are reluctant to report their pain to nurses or doctors (Brockopp *et al.*, 1998). There are several reasons why this may happen, even when we may have emphasised how important it is that they tell us about their pain.

Time out Think about why patients are likely not to report their pain to you. Make a list of possible reasons.

Some common misconceptions about pain from a patient's perspective are:

- Pain is to be expected with disease and cancer.
- I have no control over my pain.
- Opioids cause too many problems, for example constipation, sickness, sleepiness and addiction.
- I should wait as long as possible before taking a pain killer.
- The nurse knows whether I need a pain killer.
- The nurses are too busy for me to ask for a pain killer.
- If I need a higher dose of a strong pain killer, I am becoming an addict.
- It is culturally unacceptable, for example with regard to the British stiff upper lip.
- I can only have pain killers for my pain and I would prefer not to.

Minimising pain is a very real problem for some patients (and their carers), which can impede genuine attempts to manage their pain effectively. There have to date been relatively few studies exploring the patient's contribution to pain management. Many of the medical research studies assume patients to be the passive recipients of their treatment, and Reisner (1993) argues that the views of the patient have been eclipsed in medicine. He suggests this may be changing and proposes that the advent of the ethics movement and the interest in outcomes will move the views of the patients to the centre of the health care stage.

Activity

Ask a few patients whom they see as being the authority on their pain?

In the light of their comments, is there anything you would do differently?

The reasons for patients minimising their pain are outlined below.

Patients think that the nurse is the authority on their pain

If patients view you as the one who knows most about their pain, they are unlikely to share with you their true feelings; they may assume that you will know when they need analgesia. This could be further endorsed if a general question such as 'Have you any pain Mr Jones?' is asked during the drug round. Patients may assume that the nurse knows whether they needed analgesia so they are likely to refuse any unless they feel that the nurse thinks they should have some. In some situations, for example after surgery, it may be more helpful for the nurse to assume that the patient will have some pain or discomfort. Letting patients know that you expect them to have pain/discomfort may help them to tell you more about their pain. It is important to combine this with a formal pain assessment. (Refer back to Chapter 2 for examples of simple assessment tools.)

Low expectations about pain relief

Scott and Hodson (1997) surveyed 529 people attending the general practitioner about their knowledge of postoperative pain and the methods available to treat it. They found that the public had confidence in the ability of the doctors and nurses to treat this pain and little understanding of postoperative pain or the methods available to control pain. It is essential that we educate patients with regard to their pain relief, otherwise they will continue to have low expectations, which will only serve to perpetuate poor standards (Gabrielczyk, 1995).

Fear of injections

In children, the fear of needles is recognised, and the regular use of topical local anaesthetics, as well as the greater use of intravenous, intranasal and oral medication, has reduced the fear associated with injections. In the adult population this fear is largely ignored, yet many adults also fear injections. Sensitive assessment should identify individuals who fear needles and thus avoid analgesia offered via this route. Sublingual preparations and suppositories are often not offered to patients but can be just as effective.

Fear of addiction

With the current media messages conveying the dangers of drugs and addiction, coupled with health care professionals' irrational concerns with the risk of addiction (Morgan, 1985; Vortherms *et al.*, 1992), it is no wonder that the general public are reluctant to receive these drugs. Nurses may inadvertently make comments such as 'You are better off not taking the stronger ones' or 'We don't want you becoming dependent on them', which only endorse patient concerns. To add to the problem, patients, who have been on strong opioids for some time, may then experience unpleasant withdrawal symptoms if these are abruptly stopped. This is mistaken for addiction, and the unfortunate patient may then be reluctant to take such drugs again.

Implications of the pain

Patients may worry that when they start to experience pain or their pain increases, this signals the onset of disease progression, for example cancer that has spread. Denying their pain may be part of their coping strategy at this time. Another reason for minimising pain is the fear that discharge home will be delayed: patients may feel that once they are 'pain free', they will be allowed home. It would thus make sense to appear to require little or no medication and deny any discomfort. If you suspect that a patient may be minimising his or her pain, it is essential sensitively to explore the possible reason for this. Some patients feel that their pain should be tolerable because it was '*only* a hernia repair' or 'not as bad as Mrs Smith's'. It is important that staff are sensitive to these perceptions and always assess pain formally.

Activity

For each of the reasons discussed, identify how you might ensure that patients feel they can be open and honest about their pain.

Ask patients about their pain and whether they have been reluctant to report it.

Make some notes for each one.

ORGANISATIONAL ASPECTS

Fagerhaugh and Strauss (1977) looked at the organisational setting in which pain management took place and felt that the discrepancy between actual and potential pain relief might be due to the work demands in the clinical area, the lack of accountability surrounding pain management and the complexity of the patient–staff relationship. More recent studies have highlighted similar areas relating to the knowledge of health care professionals, poor working relationships and a lack of institutional resources (Brockopp *et al.*, 1998).

It has been acknowledged that legal constraints and institutional policies can unnecessarily limit nurses' ability to manage pain safely and effectively (Jacox *et al.*, 1992), but there is little research available that has identified the influence of such policies. Publications such as *The Patient's Charter* (DoH, 1991) provide the patient with a stronger voice in practice and may act as a lever to improve pain control. The setting and implementation of minimum standards and the effects of clinical governance may also drive improvements in the way in which we manage pain in the future. A number of initiatives will provide the catalyst for these changes; multidisciplinary working, partnerships with patients and users and increased use of evidence-based practice. (NHSE, 1999).

Formal documents and policies can be a catalyst to improve pain management, a good example of this being the Royal College of Surgeons and the College of Anaesthetists (1990) *Report of the Working Party on Pain after Surgery*. This document resulted in many hospitals forming acute pain teams (see Chapter 3). Let us look now at some of these assumptions in more detail.

WORK DEMANDS IN THE CLINICAL AREA

There is no doubt that the pace of work has considerably increased in recent years. Contributing factors such as shortened hospital stay, increased longevity and diminishing resources are implicated. Nurses are busy, doctors are busy, everyone is very busy. Most patients hesitate to trouble staff for fear of being regarded as a nuisance (Winefield *et al.*, 1990). Carr and Thomas (1997) found that patients' unwillingness to trouble staff, even when they were in pain, was a major barrier to obtaining effective pain relief.

Activity

How could you create an environment that oozed a feeling of timelessness in order to encourage patients to stop and ask you for pain relief?

This is not easy, but it is worth a try.

Creating a relaxing environment is not always easy, especially when you are busy. Gentle instrumental music in the background and the use of plants can provide a feeling of calm. Try to maintain eye contact with patients, and always ask open questions regarding their pain. Questions such as 'Tell me about your pain' encourage patients to share their experience with you and suggest to them that you are interested and have time to listen.

Lack of accountability

Although each nurse is held accountable for his or her actions (UKCC, 1992), the issue about accountability in pain management is not easily resolved. If pain management is not effective who is to blame? Some may say the doctor did not prescribe the appropriate medication; another might suggest that the nurses did not administer the analgesia regularly enough. Some hospitals may have an acute pain service, and accountability may be seen to be vested in the 'team'. Similarly, accountability for cancer pain management in the community may be seen to lie with the Macmillan team. Nursing staff can be in a key position to be accountable for pain management. They often care for an individual 24 hours a day, and they are the central co-ordinators for the input of other health care professionals, but do we see ourselves as accountable? Nurses will have a key role to play in the development of clinical governance (Moores, 1999). Improving accountability for the management of pain will be an important part of these endeavours.

Time out Think about someone you have cared for whose pain was well managed. Who was accountable for their pain management? Now ask some colleagues (including those from other professions) who is accountable for a patient's pain management.

The importance of accountability

Lack of accountability has been implicated as a key factor contributing to ineffective pain management (Lander, 1990). You probably found difficulty in identifying one person who held accountability. Some may see the consultant physician as being 'accountable', but does this help when he or she might see the patient only every 3 days? If the nurse is seen as accountable, but unable to prescribe, this might also present difficulties. There is no clear-cut answer, but nurses have a central role to play as they are the continuous link between health professionals.

The organisation of nursing care and approaches such as 'primary nursing' and the 'named nurse' concept can do much to enhance accountability. Primary nursing has at its centre concepts such as advocacy, accountability and individualised care (Pearson, 1988). The delivery of care will continue to change, and initiatives such as 'clinical governance' will continue to shape the provision of pain management, increasingly putting pressure on health care staff to deliver an improved quality of care. Questions about effectiveness and measurement will act as a catalyst for organisations to evaluate their pain management, and some are doing so already. More patient-centred health care delivery, which is modern and dependable, is the philosophy of *The New National Health Service* (DoH, 1998), and health care professionals and senior management will be held increasingly accountable for the delivery of acceptable, humane and knowledgeable practice.

Institutional policies

The requirement of most hospitals for two nurses to check a controlled drug can increase the length of time over which patients suffer pain, and reducing this to single-nurse administration would considerably speed up the delivery of analgesia. Registered nurses dispensing drugs alone currently give far more lethal drugs, for example digoxin, without checking with another practitioner. Similarly, hospital policy may not allow controlled drugs to be dispensed from the drug trolley, although this could be challenged. The ability to give an oral opioid from the drug trolley could significantly reduce the time that patients would wait in pain for the nurse to come back with the analgesia. Although it is over 10 years old, an informative chapter by White (1985) raises a number of issues regarding hospital policy and pain control. Clinicians should be encouraged to challenge hospital policies that mitigate against effective pain management. The ability critically to consider the environment one practices in is nothing more than professional, and if policies are found that may contribute to ineffective pain management, they should be challenged.

Research summary

- A study was undertaken in 1995 to examine the time taken to administer controlled drugs (CDs) in a hospice (with seven beds)
- A stopwatch was used to measure the time from the decision to administer a CD to its administration (two trained nurses being available)
- The annual cost of administering CDs was £10,883.94
- The annual cost of the CDs was £3647.31
- Administration accounted for 75 per cent of the total cost
- Recommendation: **AVOID USING CONTROLLED DRUGS**

McGettrick and Rogers (1996)

Activity

Reflect on the findings from this study.

Could anything else have been done to reduce the cost of administering the controlled drugs?

What effect might the recommendation from this study have on pain management on this hospice ward?

Solutions that avoid tackling organisational policies can be very short-term approaches. In this situation, such a change in practice could reduce effective pain management. Another approach might have been to discuss the findings with the Director of Nursing. If the problems and possible solutions have been well thought out and evidence of a need for change obtained, it is often extremely satisfying to challenge traditional practice and bring about change that can have far-reaching benefits for patients. Single nurse administration is a good example.

LIMITATIONS OF PRESCRIBING

All too often, short-acting intramuscular analgesia is prescribed on a prn basis instead of prescribing regular 'balanced analgesia' to maintain pain relief. A prn prescription tends to ensure that the patient with an ongoing painful condition, which may last for days, experiences a return of pain before asking for further analgesia. Patients may even be eating and drinking, but the intramuscular route is still maintained. By prescribing a range of analgesic drugs, for example an opioid combined with an NSAID or paracetamol, matched to the patient's need, titrated to the patient's response and reviewed on a regular basis, far better analgesia can be maintained (McQuay *et al.*, 1997).

It is likely that documents such as the Crown Report (1999) will facilitate vast changes in the laws governing the nurse's role in the administration of drugs. Group protocols will enable nurses to administer certain analgesia immediately without a prescription.

INTERPROFESSIONAL PAIN EDUCATION

The inadequate knowledge of health care professionals is one of the most prevalent causative factors in studies documenting the under-treatment of pain (Greipp, 1992; Clarke *et al.*, 1996). The majority of nurse education undergraduate programmes include pain management in the curriculum, but the average of just 4 hours of study does not prepare students adequately (Graffam, 1990). As previously mentioned, Marcer and Deighton (1988) highlighted the problem of little or no pain education for medical students, with scant evidence of multidisciplinary teaching.

Funnell (1995) reviewed the literature and identified four expected outcomes associated with shared learning. Understanding the roles and perceptions of other professionals, and the promotion of future teamwork, leads to co-operation between professional groups. This in turn contributes to enhancing the learner's knowledge base and the development of practical skills.

The term 'interprofessional' suggests shared learning, which aims to help professionals to work together more effectively in the interests of their patients by enhancing co-operation and collaboration (Michaud, 1970). Interprofessional pain education should explicitly link to the everyday world of clinical practice; for example, if the prescribed analgesia is not relieving the pain, the nurse needs the knowledge and skills to negotiate a change in the prescription. Education must address the knowledge, skills and confidence required to deliver effective pain management in a multiprofessional environment.

A questionnaire was given to all teachers in Finnish medical faculties in 1991 and 1995 (Poyhia and Kalso, 1999), using the International Association for the Study of Pain (IASP) curricula to evaluate and compare with current teaching. The results were very disappointing, revealing no printed curriculum in any university, and the picture had not changed between 1991 and 1995. A serious lack of time allotted to psychology of pain was found within the teaching. Recommendations were made to focus on changing the attitudes of the university teachers to pain, that the IASP should distribute curricula to the governing bodies of the universities and that a multimedia teaching package be produced to accompany the curricula.

Activity

How could you promote interprofessional pain education in your practice?

A study day would be one way of providing an opportunity for different professionals to come together and learn about pain, but time constraints and resources are often prohibitive. It might be possible to build pain education into some activities that already involve different professionals coming together, for example for a case conference or ward round. Having 15 minutes to discuss a particular patient and his or her pain management can encourage professionals to share their viewpoints and problem-solve. Alternatively, sharing a research paper and discussing it informally can get people thinking differently about pain management in their clinical area.

IMPROVING PRACTICE

case history

The nurses in a small palliative care team were expressing their frustration at trying to manage a patient's pain that was not responding to the prescribed analgesia. The patient might have to wait a considerable time if the doctor was busy in the accident and emergency department at the other side of the hospital. The doctors and nurses discussed possible solutions to the problem and came up with the idea of ensuring that pain was assessed before 8 a.m. A protocol could be drawn up to cover the administration of 'one off' analgesia in certain situations, and a list of non-pharmacological strategies could be utilised to help the patient in the interim period. The discussion led the nurses to reflect on how pain was currently assessed and managed. They realised that if a patient's pain had been closely monitored, it was unlikely that this situation would occur.

The simplest of strategies can be the most effective and often arise when just a few interested professionals manage to take the time to discuss what could be improved and how to improve it.

CONCLUSION

Barriers to effective pain management present unique challenges to practitioners. Education is probably the most important tool for improving pain management (Lander, 1990). There is, however, a need to develop innovative multiprofessional education so that health care professionals can collaboratively facilitate change in their environment, be prepared to develop lifelong learning and utilise research-based knowledge in their practice.

Future changes in health care will bring increased pressure for better pain management. The hospital treatment of patients is likely to result in sicker, more dependent individuals being nursed in general wards rather than high-dependency units. Early discharge home and increased day case surgery, as well as a larger number of elderly clients, will increase the prevalence of pain in the community. It is essential that practitioners are armed with the most appropriate pain knowledge and can critically consider potential barriers to effective pain management.

After a break, try the multiple-choice questionnaire below in order to self-assess your learning so far.

Suggested further reading

Dufault, M.A., Bielecki, C., Collins, E. and Wiley, C. (1995) Changing nurses' pain assessment practice: a collaborative research utilization approach. *Journal of Advanced Nursing*, **21**: 634–45.

Fordham, M. and Dunn, V. (1994) *Alongside the Person in Pain. Holistic Care and Nursing Practice*, London, Baillière Tindall. (See Chapter 8.)

Francke, A.L. and Theeuwen, I. (1994) Inhibition in expression of pain: a qualitative study among Dutch surgical breast cancer patients. *Cancer Nursing*, **17**(3): 193–9.

Hawthorn, J. and Redmond, K. (1998) *Pain Causes and Management*, Oxford, Blackwell Science. (See Chapter 5.)

Thomas, N.V. (ed.) (1997) *Pain: Its Nature and Management*, London, Baillière Tindall.

Salerno, E. and Willens, J. (eds) *Pain Management: Handbook: An Interdisciplinary Approach*, St Louis, C.V. Mosby.

Watt-Watson, J.H. and Donovan, M.I. (1992) *Pain Management: Nursing Perspective*, St Louis, Mosby Year Book. (See Chapter 3.)

Wilkie, D., Williams, A.R., Grevstad, P. and Mekwa, J. (1995) Coaching persons with lung cancer to report sensory pain. *Cancer Nursing*, **18**(1): 7–15.

Barriers to Effective Pain Relief

MULTIPLE-CHOICE QUESTIONNAIRE

1. Which factor has been identified as the most important cause of inadequate pain management?

   a. Cultural beliefs ☐

   b. Inadequate assessment ☐

   c. Misconceptions ☐

   d. Lack of knowledge ☐

2. Which of the following statements is true?

   a. Patients experiencing pain do not always report their pain accurately ☐

   b. Chronic pain is not as serious as acute pain ☐

   c. Patients should expect to experience pain in hospital ☐

   d. Patients will always tell you when they have pain ☐

3. Which statement best reflects why patients may minimise their pain?

   a. Analgesics are harmful ☐

   b. It is important to feel pain so I won't overdo it ☐

   c. Pain is to be expected and the nurse will know whether I am in pain ☐

   d. The nurses will be pleased with me if I say that I have no pain ☐

MULTIPLE-CHOICE QUESTIONNAIRE (cont'd)

4. Misconceptions held by health care professionals can contribute to ineffective pain relief. The fears surrounding opioids are well documented. Which statement is true?

   a. Regular opioids for 2 weeks result in 30 per cent of patients becoming addicted ☐

   b. Regular opioids for 2 weeks result in 60 per cent of patients becoming addicted ☐

   c. It is not possible to predict the chances of someone becoming addicted ☐

   d. Regular opioids for 2 weeks result in a less than 1 per cent of patients becoming addicted ☐

5. Which statement might not discourage a patient from accepting an opioid for pain relief?

   a. You don't want to get dependent on them ☐

   b. You are better off not taking them if you don't want to ☐

   c. Patients say that they would prefer not to take them and the nurse praises them ☐

   d. It is important to keep you comfortable so that you move and cough regularly ☐

6. Most patients hesitate to trouble staff for fear of being:

   a. Too popular ☐   c. Boring ☐

   b. A nuisance ☐   d. Ignored ☐

7. The organisation can inhibit effective pain management as a result of:

   a. A lack of accountability on the part of health care professionals ☐

   b. Not having clear patterns of communication ☐

   c. A lack of quiet periods in the clinical area ☐

   d. A lack of hospital policies that encourage effective pain management ☐

8. Which of the following might increase accountability for pain?

   a. Team nursing ☐

   b. Task nursing ☐

   c. Primary nursing ☐

   d. Patient allocation ☐

9. Which is the most important tool for improving pain management?

   a. More nursing staff ☐

   b. Education ☐

   c. A wider range of analgesics ☐

   d. Nurse prescribing ☐

MULTIPLE-CHOICE QUESTIONNAIRE (cont'd)

10. Which approach to the provision of education on pain management is likely to have the most impact on practice?

   a. Formal lectures in a classroom for nurses of all grades ☐

   b. Lunch-time discussions around a 'patient', involving all professionals ☐

   c. Discussions on the ward rounds ☐

   d. Planned multidisciplinary teaching around a patient case study ☐

ANSWERS FOR THE MULTIPLE-CHOICE QUESTIONNAIRE

1.   d. **Lack of knowledge** of health care professionals was cited most often in the studies reporting inadequate pain management (Griepp, 1992).

2.   a. **Patients experiencing pain do not always report their pain accurately;** there are numerous reasons why patients might minimise their pain: not wanting to be a bother to the nurses, anxiety about pain delaying their return home, wanting to appear stoic or feeling that it is unacceptable to show that they have pain.

3.   c. **Pain is to be expected and the nurse will know whether I am in pain;** many patients believe that pain is to be expected and have low expectations regarding the management of their pain. Research has shown that patients will expect the nurse to know when they have pain, but nurses might expect patients to *tell* them if they have pain. These factors are powerful inhibitors of effective pain management. It should be noted that the other statements may also prevent patients expressing their pain.

4.   d. **Regular opioids for 2 weeks results in a less than 1 per cent of patients becoming addicted.**

5.   d. **It is important to keep you comfortable so that you move and cough regularly**; this statement informs the patients why it is important to remain comfortable; this is likely to encourage them to accept analgesia. The remaining statements would all encourage patients to refuse analgesia.

6.   b. **A nuisance.**

7.   a. **Lack of accountability on the part of health care professionals** has been reported as one of the reasons why there is a discrepancy between actual and potential pain relief in the clinical area. Fagerhaugh and Strauss (1977) suggest that high work demands and rigid hospital policies may also contribute. Communication is also important but accountability would help this as well.

8.   c. **Primary nursing** focuses on individualised nursing care, one nurse being responsible for the care of a particular patient. This would facilitate accurate pain

assessment and individual accountability. The other methods of care delivery have less structured forms of accountability.

9. b. **Education** is suggested to be the remedy for the evident lack of knowledge in studies that report an inadequate management of pain. It is unlikely that more nursing staff, nurse prescribing and a wider range of analgesics will have much impact unless those involved have the knowledge to utilise them effectively.

10. d. **Planned multidisciplinary teaching around a patient case study** offers all those professionals involved in the patient's pain management the chance to participate together. They are likely to share the difficulties they have encountered, which can be invaluable in promoting effective communication and learning from their experiences. Lunch-time discussions can be a good second best. Formal lectures may not address the difficulties encountered in practice. Ward rounds can be useful, but time and issues of privacy might inhibit fruitful learning.

6 Managing pain in vulnerable patients

LEARNING OUTCOMES

On completion of this chapter the student will be able to:

■ Discuss patient groups that are particularly vulnerable to inadequate pain assessment and management

■ Identify a pain assessment strategy for a vulnerable patient and discuss the rationale for the choice

■ Analyse factors that might contribute to the inadequate management of pain for these patient groups

■ Evaluate strategies that might lead to improved pain relief

INDICATIVE READING

Baker, A., Bowring, L., Brignell, A. and Kafford, D. (1996) Chronic pain management in cognitively impaired patients: a preliminary research project. *Perspectives*, **20**(2): 4–8.

Bates, M.S., Edwards, W.T. and Anderson, K.O. (1993) Ethnocultural influences on variation in chronic pain perception. *Pain*, **52**: 101–12.

Cate, J.J., Morse, J.M. and James, S.G. (1991) The pain response of the post-operative newborn. *Journal of Advanced Nursing*, **16**: 378–87.

Donovan, J. (1997) Pain signals. *Nursing Times*, **93**(45): 60–2.

Finley, G.A. and McGrath P.J. (eds) (1998) *Measurement of Pain in Infants and Children*, Seattle, IASP Press.

Hayes, L. (1997) A cultural experience of pain, In Moore, S. (ed.) *Understanding Pain and its Relief in Labour*, Edinburgh, Churchill Livingstone, Chapter 6. (for midwifery students.)

Horgan, M., Choonara, I., Al-Waidh, M., Sambrooks, J. and Ashby, D. (1996) Measuring pain in neonates: an objective score. *Paediatric Nursing*, **8**(10): 24–7.

McGrath, P.J., Rosmus, C., Canfield, C., Campbell, M.A. and Hennigar, A. (1998) Behaviours caregivers use to determine pain in non-verbal, cognitively impaired individuals. *Developmental Medicine and Child Neurology*, **40**(5): 340–3.

Moddeman, G.R. (1995) Barriers to pain management in elderly surgical patients. *AORN Journal*, **61**(6): 1073–5.

Simons, W. and Malabar, R. (1995) Assessing pain in elderly patients who cannot respond verbally. *Journal of Advanced Nursing*, **22**(4): 663–9.

BACKGROUND

If you look through the current literature on the assessment and management of pain, the vast majority of it assumes that the pain is experienced by patients who can communicate verbally. Being able to communicate effectively makes the assessment and treatment of pain relatively straightforward: you and your patient can join together as a team to experiment with interventions, and to evaluate their efficacy using a variety of well-tested assessment tools. For some patients, however, the ability to communicate may be absent, impaired or not yet developed. Alternatively, cultural and language differences may hamper adequate assessment and treatment. For all such people, you will find the literature scant, to say the least. Drawing on our own experiences and the literature that does exist, we have assembled some of the key points for providing pain relief for vulnerable people.

Activity

Carry out a brief literature search to identify articles on pain management in a particularly vulnerable client group.

Do you notice any gaps or difficulties?

Why do you think this might be?

'Vulnerable' is defined in the dictionary as 'capable of being physically or emotionally wounded or hurt', the thesaurus listing alternative descriptions such as 'defenceless, exposed, susceptible, unprotected and weak' (Collins, 1987). An editorial in *Nursing Clinics of North America* begins by stating:

> Vulnerable populations are social groups who experience relatively more illness, premature death, and diminished quality of life than comparable groups. Vulnerable populations are often poor; many are discriminated against or subordinated; and they are frequently marginalized and disenfranchised. Vulnerable populations typically include women and children, ethnic people of colour, immigrants, the homeless, the elderly, and gay men and women. (Flaskerud, 1999, pp. xv–xvi)

In particular, we shall be looking at how communication difficulties are the principal factors that render these patients vulnerable or susceptible to hurt through the inadequate recognition and treatment of their pain.

You will probably find that the more vulnerable your patient group, the less has been written or researched on the subject of their pain management. In fact, Liebeskind and Melzack (1987) have said that 'pain is most poorly managed in those who are most defenceless against it'. This is probably because it is particularly difficult not only to assess this group of patients, but also to find and evaluate a therapy that will provide the optimum response for the fewest side-effects.

Activity

Skim the index and some of the chapters of a pain textbook to see whether attention is paid to vulnerable people.

What do you notice?

If pain management is mentioned in this context, do the books stress the 'difficulty', or do they give practical help on how to manage or approach specific problems? More often than not, no mention is made of these groups. Admittedly, these patients can baffle us with the complexity of their needs, but providing adequate analgesia is not impossible, as we shall see later from some case histories.

Before we go any further, it might be useful to define some of the vulnerable patient groups that this chapter will discuss. We should stress that the list of groups identified is not exhaustive, but we aim to cover a wide selection of people. We shall be looking at the needs of the *cognitively impaired*, whether their state has arisen as the result of age-related Alzheimer's disease or senile dementia, as a consequence of severe learning disabilities, or following a stoke or trauma that has led to brain damage. We shall also be looking at the needs of *unconscious patients* and *neonates*, and the problems associated with communication with *small children*. In addition, we shall briefly consider some of the work that has been done with patients from different *ethnic backgrounds*, who may encounter language problems, who may be unable to convey their thoughts and feelings to staff from a different culture, or for whom pain has a meaning different from our own. These are of course not the only groups of patient who have traditionally experienced inadequate pain management as a result of communication problems, misconception, knowledge deficit or even prejudice.

Chapter 7 will investigate the pain management needs of challenging patients, those with psychosocial or behavioural problems, complex pathologies or a history of substance abuse.

Time out   List the patients whom you can think of who have suffered inadequate pain assessment/management. What do you consider were the difficulties of pain management for each of them?

DEFINING THE BARRIERS

When you have collected the information, try to summarise your findings. Putting the answers into a table format can be helpful. Preparing a matrix like the one in Table 6.1 may help you to categorise the

Table 6.1   Matrix for identifying barriers to effective pain management

CLIENT GROUPS:	Brain injured	Learning disabilities	Elderly	Dementia, for example Alzheimer's	Small children	Ethnic minorities	Others
PROBLEMS: Communication problems							
Misconceptions							
Knowledge deficit							
Compliance problems							
Absence of assessment tools							
Institutional barriers							
Political barriers							
Others – specify							

various problems that may be encountered by each client group. These can then be linked to see where problems are specific or where they are shared by particular groups of patients.

Having carried out this exercise, you may now be clearer in your own mind as to what particular difficulties your patient groups may encounter. All the above patients present significant challenges, but each group has specific areas of difficulty. You may have come up with an even longer list of patients who are particularly vulnerable. However, having completed this exercise, it may now be useful to look at each of the groups we have listed above individually. We can then attempt to expand on the specific barriers that might obstruct their pain management. Once we are aware of the problems we face, we shall then be in a better position to devise solutions.

PAIN IN THE ELDERLY

 Evidence strongly suggests that pain and cognitive impairment may coexist in a high proportion of older persons. As Parmelee (1996) states, 'the management of either problem alone is a challenge; their concurrence may well test the limits of the skills of professional and informal caregivers alike'. With an increasingly older population, it is essential that we develop the knowledge and skills to manage pain in this group of people effectively.

Some facts and figures

One study revealed that, from a sample of nursing home and day care patients, 83 per cent experienced pain (Roy and Thomas, 1986). Marzinski (1991) reported that 70 per cent of nursing home residents indicated that they had pain and 34 per cent constant pain, while 66 per cent reported intermittent pain. Despite the prevalence of pain, only 15 per cent of the patients had received any analgesia in the previous 24 hours. A publication by Crombie *et al.* (1999) provides vital, up-to-date epidemiological information for those wishing further information on the prevalence and incidence of pain.

One of the first problems to tackle is that of pain assessment. Go into any areas that deal with the care of the elderly, whether or not cognitively impaired and given the extent of the problem, doesn't it strike you as odd that temperature and pulse may be recorded regularly but it is doubtful that you will find a similar record of regular pain assessment? Although regular pain assessment is inappropriate for patients suffering chronic or intractable pain, this may even be the case when the pain is of an acute and therefore eminently treatable nature.

PAIN MANAGEMENT IN THE COGNITIVELY IMPAIRED ELDERLY PATIENT

There is unfortunately very little research examining the ability of health care professionals or family members to estimate pain in the cognitively impaired person, although there is some research to indicate that, so far, we have all been doing rather badly. Health care professionals appear to be particularly poor at pain estimation, the bulk of the evidence tending to show an underestimation of pain intensity (Choiniere *et al.*, 1990). Dementia or brain injury and its consequent problems, such as impaired formal thinking, lead to the formation of less sophisticated concepts of pain. This may then cause painful pathology to be masked by or missed altogether because of behavioural disturbances (Corran and Melita, 1998). Perhaps more alarming is the fact that when health care professionals do recognise that pain is probably present, they fail to prescribe and administer analgesia as they would for those patients able to communicate (Sengstaken and King, 1993). What is it like in your area?

Activity

What percentage of your patients do you think experience regular pain?

During one shift, ask each elderly patient who can communicate verbally whether he or she experiences pain on a regular basis.

Given that you were only asking those patients able to communicate their pain, what percentage of elderly patients overall do you now think experience regular pain?

We are sure you will find that pain in the elderly is a major problem in your clinical area, but it is usually underrecognised. Now you have ascertained the extent of pain in this population, it is probably safe to estimate that the prevalence of pain is pretty much the same for those unable to express their pain verbally. However, as Parmelee (1996) concluded, there could well be an association between cognitive impairment and a decreased propensity to report pain even when it is present. Farrell *et al.* (1996) noted less reporting of pain by cognitively impaired people and even less in those significantly impaired.

Growing older may not necessarily mean pain and disability as the majority of older adults lead a healthy and active life. Some diseases, for example arthritis, are, however, more prevalent in an older population. It is estimated that rheumatoid arthritis affects over 5 per cent of women over 65 years old (Hawthorn and Redmond, 1998) and osteoarthritis about 10 per cent of the population, although it is principally associated with ageing (Dieppe, 1987). People with a pain-eliciting pathology may well be very accepting of their discomfort and 'lot in life', and have a low expectation for relief; similarly, health care professionals may accept that pain is inevitable and to be accepted. This should not, however, be the case.

Other conditions usually associated with ageing may contribute to pain. Gibson and Helme (1995) pointed out that fewer than 25 per cent of individuals remain disability-free by the age of 70 years and fewer than 15 per cent by the age of 80. You may be able to think of a considerable list of conditions associated with ageing that blight the enjoyment of retirement and give rise to a slower pace of life. Table 6.2 may help to highlight some of the more common potential causes of pain.

Osteoarthritis, post-herpetic neuralgia and post-stroke pain are rare in the young but account for 60 per cent of the patients attending the pain clinic for the elderly in Melbourne, Australia (Helme *et al.*, 1989).

Most elderly patients may, to a greater or lesser extent, display one or a combination of the above problems. Farrell *et al.* (1996) provided a summary of epidemiological studies in the elderly, which indicated that non-malignant pain was a common experience. For patients who can communicate their pain there is no reason why pain cannot be assessed and strategies selected to ameliorate their suffering. For those who cannot communicate effectively, it is up to us to ensure that if a painful condition exists, we are aware of it. We then need to be more creative in our approach to the assessment and management of these patients' pain.

Table 6.2   Types of disease and potential pain

Source	Type of pain
Arthritis	Joint pain, especially in large joints such as the hips and knees: the prevalence of this type of pain is more than doubled in older adults compared with younger people (Gibson and Helme, 1995). Low back pain, neck pain
Cancer	The prevalence of cancer increases with age. Disease progression may lead to nerve compression, pain from bony metastasis, raised intracranial pressure, visceral pain, lymphoedema, treatment such as neuropathic damage following radiotherapy, postoperative pain following surgery, or drugs causing nausea, constipation or sore mouth
Diabetes	Nerve damage pain from peripheral neuropathy, tissue damage, ulcers
Cardiovascular system	Angina, intermittent claudication of the legs, venous leg ulcers, post-stroke pain
Virus infection	Post-herpetic neuralgia, complex regional pain syndrome
Musculoskeletal complaints	Osteoporosis causing fractures and contractures, complex regional pain syndrome
Multiple diseases	Combinations of all or some of the above

Where verbal communication is not possible, non-verbal behaviours should be considered. Nurses need to observe non-verbal cues, such as facial expression and gross motor behaviour, in order to assess pain. We now have plenty of research on non-verbal expressions of pain in cognitively intact patients of all ages, which tend to show consistency in both facial and 'body language' indicators of pain. Perhaps these indicators can be adapted for use in your area to help to develop some sort of behavioural pain assessment tool.

Activity

Choose three cognitively impaired elderly patients whom you consider could be in pain.

These patients could be suffering dementia from a variety of causes, for example Alzheimer's disease.

Are you able to identify certain behaviours that you feel may consistently indicate the presence of pain?

Moaning	Aggressive
Outgoing	Noisy breathing
Quiet	Friendly
Agitated	Rocking
Cheerful	Disjointed verbalisation
Withdrawn	Involved
Mute	Eats well
Verbally abusive	Describes pain
Cries easily	Calling out
Refuses food	Picking

(Baker et al., 1996)

Figure 6.1 Behaviours that help to indicate pain

If you have worked in long-term health care settings, or indeed any setting where pain is not easily relieved, you will probably have observed many behaviours that appear to be associated with pain. Baker *et al.* (1996) adapted Frank *et al.*'s (1992) Facial Grimace Scale and a behaviour checklist (Marzinski, 1991), which showed promising results. Figure 6.1 lists the behaviours they identified to help to assess pain and discomfort.

These observations may provide you with the basis for developing or adapting a pain assessment tool. In the past, doubt has been cast on the reliability of observed behaviours because of patients' differing coping styles and social and cultural backgrounds, as well as the impact of anxiety and depression (Closs, 1994). However, it appears that observations can be matched quite well with Keefe and Block's (1982) five-category system of non-verbal approaches to pain assessment. This system relies on observing *guarding, bracing, rubbing, grimacing* and *sighing*. Observing these behaviours has already been adapted for use with cancer patients by Ahles *et al.* (1984); patients suffering from rheumatoid arthritis by Anderson *et al.* (1992); and recently by Simons and Malabar (1995) specifically for pain in elderly patients unable to respond verbally.

Time out   Having identified some of the behaviours you might observe, how
would you measure them?
What sort of criteria would you use?

Measurement scales for observation can be devised by using simple categories such as 'none', 'a little' or 'a lot'. Although these seem quite straightforward, they are not always reliable as they require the subjective judgement of the observer. One person might judge 'a little' to be the same as another's 'a lot'. To avoid discrepancy between the different assessors, it is helpful to have some sort of quantitative measure, for example 'none' = 0, 'a little' = 1–5 and 'a lot' = 6–10. A description to verify the score makes the judgement less subject to bias and can be particularly helpful.

case history

Mrs B is admitted to an orthopaedic ward from a residential care home with a fractured neck of femur. She has a longstanding history of dementia and no close relatives, and there has been little liaison between the nursing home and the orthopaedic ward staff. Prior to her surgery, Mrs B seemed quiet and withdrawn.

Several hours after returning from theatre following a hip replacement, Mrs B becomes noisy and obviously distressed. She is given an intramuscular opioid and settles rapidly. Two hours later, she is once again noisy and distressed. No formal pain assessment has been commenced, the only documentation stating the fact that she received some analgesia 2 hours previously. Her analgesia is prescribed 4–6-hourly, with no prn therapy for breakthrough pain and no adjuvant therapy in the form of regular non-steroidal anti-inflammatory drugs. For the next hour, Mrs B becomes progressively noisier and disturbs the other patients. She is given a sedative and eventually quietens down. Over a period of 24 hours, this pattern is repeated, a sedative being administered on a regular basis. A senior nurse then commences an 'observed behaviour pain assessment chart' based on Mrs B's level of restlessness, noise and distress. The nurse also suggests that diclofenac and paracetamol be given on a regular basis, with oral morphine prescribed hourly on a prn basis. The change in Mrs B is immediate and positive.

Poor pain management had changed Mrs B from her normally quiet, seemingly content but somewhat withdrawn self to someone showing behaviour that was noisy, disruptive and very distressed. Once adequate pain assessment had been introduced and analgesia administered, based on the findings from this assessment, the patient changed back to her usual self. She required no further sedation and went on to regain her previous mobility. Through a rehabilitation programme, she was discharged to her home a week later.

You might think that the above scenario is uncommon and that elderly patients are never left to suffer pain. Unfortunately, however, the evidence suggests that Mrs B's earlier treatment is far from rare. Wall and Jones (1991) provide a summary of a case that occurred in 1988 in a National Health Service teaching hospital in which a frail elderly woman in severe pain from a fractured femur was ignored. Her cries disturbed other patients so she was moved to a dark side room with no bell or light switch. This was not necessarily the behaviour of a callous, uncaring nurse. Referral to Chapter 5 highlights the problems associated with the poor prescribing habits of medical staff, the non-existence of pain assessment, misconceptions surrounding the use of powerful analgesia and the bureaucratic barriers that can sometimes leave nurses feeling powerless to remedy a situation in which they only play a part.

How could Mrs B's initial situation have been avoided? Would it have been useful to ask the carers at Mrs B's home or her relatives about her normal behaviour? They may be able to provide useful information about what a particular behaviour might indicate, whether the patient normally responds to pain or discomfort in this way and what the possible causes of pain may be when they are not as blindingly obvious as a fractured femur. They can also provide information about what may have been a useful treatment in the past and how the patient coped with pain and discomfort if and when he or she was able to communicate. Using an 'around-the-clock' prescription for analgesia might have avoided some of the problems. All these strategies will help you to devise a way of assessing and managing pain more effectively with the cognitively impaired elderly person.

A pain diary that stays with patients and can be taken with them when they change environments could be invaluable. It could be used by staff or relatives to document any pain management strategies that have been successful, or less so, in the past, as well as any adverse effects that the therapy may have produced. Pain in the confused elderly is so often overlooked or dismissed. It would seem that, like neonates, many confused elderly patients have suffered from the assumption that they cannot feel pain, or staff feel concerned about giving them analgesia unnecessarily. This should not be the case. A trial period of analgesia and regular documentation of their pain behaviour is an effective way of assessing analgesic requirements. Remember too that mild pain can respond very well to other strategies, such as comfort, touch, massage, warm baths, heat pads and distraction.

LEARNING DISABILITY AND BRAIN-INJURED PATIENTS

The difficulties encountered for patients with any cognitive impairment are similar to those of elderly patients suffering from some form of dementia. However, the care of brain-injured patients can highlight some added challenges that have to be considered. The difficulties associated with their care will depend on their degree of disability and handicap. As with the elderly, various descriptors have been used to guide their care and assessment. Significant correlations were found when these descriptors were modified to assess pain in another group of patients in whom self-reported pain was matched to head and trunk tenseness, guarding/holding, rubbing, appearing drawn, squinting, grunting and sighing (Teske *et al.*, 1983).

While the self-report, however limited, will always be the 'gold standard' for pain assessment, other methods of pain assessment can be successful, especially when staff and relatives are able to identify patients' unique ways of expressing pain, sometimes in the face of severe disability. With the brain injured and those with severe learning disabilities, the key to successful treatment will hinge on being able to establish what their normal pre-pain behaviour was like and then, as with the elderly confused patient, listing those changes in behaviour that appear to be associated with pain.

NEONATES AND PREVERBAL CHILDREN

Not only do neonates lack the ability to communicate, but small children also experience communication problems. As a group, their pain management needs have probably, until very recently, been the most neglected of all (Jerrett, 1985). It is only during the past decade or so that our ignorance and widespread misconceptions about neonatal and early childhood neurological development have been challenged.

For years, it was felt that neonates and infants did not feel pain as their neuroanatomy and neurochemistry were immature. Research is now indicating that the reverse may well be the case, that because of the immaturity of pain-modulating systems, these especially vulnerable patient groups may actually experience more pain than adults. Contrary to previous thinking, there is good evidence that neonates exhibit behavioural, physiological and hormonal responses to pain (Franck, 1986). In fact, research indicated that although fetal sensory nerve fibres are complete by about the twentieth week of fetal development, the development of the endorphin and the inhibitory systems in the descending pain pathways may not be completely functional until term, making preterm infants more sensitive to pain than term infants (Fitzgerald and Koltzenburg, 1986).

Activity

Ask three colleagues what they consider to be the difficulties associated with pain management for neonates and preverbal small children.

Now that you are perhaps more aware of what you and your colleagues perceive to be some of the problems associated with pain management in small children, it will be useful to look around and see how other people facing similar challenges have responded. Good practice is so often shared only via journal articles or during conferences and is not, therefore, readily available or adequately disseminated to ward staff. The appointment of a link nurse, or utilising the expertise of staff on specialist courses, is often overlooked or undervalued. Developing a journal group to peruse the relevant literature and obtain copies for other staff members to read is also a good way of passing on good practice.

Activity

Have a quick scan through the literature to see whether you can find any of the assessment tools being developed for the management of pain in neonates.

Could any of them be adapted for your patients?

You will probably find from your last activity that, as with the elderly, the difficulties we face when trying to assess pain experienced by patients who are non-verbal can be complex. The situation is compounded by the fact that pain assessment tools developed and validated for neonates and small children are few and far between. We now seem to have plenty of assessment tools for use with verbal children that rely on their self-reporting of pain, the evidence suggesting these are useful in children of 4 years and older (Tarbel *et al.*, 1992). However, the lack of assessment tools for the very young is compounded by the anxieties that health care professionals foster about the use of opioids in this group of patients. The lack of evaluation of therapy and our inability to quantify the efficacy of analgesic techniques has led to much frustration. The situation is, however, slowly changing, and it would appear that the development of valid, research-based assessment tools for neonates and very small children is an area currently attracting some attention.

Many groups have recently been studying different aspects of neonatal behaviour in order to assess pain. Like the studies on the elderly, these have concentrated on body movement, facial expression and, in some cases, physiological responses as measures of distress. Although currently time-consuming and somewhat unwieldy, these assessments show promise. Striving for valid assessment tools is vital if we are to combat the stress response to pain in the neonate and the deleterious effect that this may have on their recovery.

Horgan *et al.* (1996) in Liverpool have described the development of a scoring system to categorise distress using eight behavioural categories, each with a 0–5 score. Termed LIDS – the Liverpool Infant Distress Score – it is based on the behaviours listed in Figure 6.2.

This study shows exciting possibilities for the future, but it can be seen from Figure 6.3 that, in order to ensure reliability, the scoring system for just one aspect alone is initially fairly long and complex.

A slightly less complex system is CRIES by Krechel and Bilner (1995) (see Table 6.3).

Spontaneous movement	Facial expression
Spontaneous excitability	Cry quality
Flexion of fingers and toes	Cry quantity
Tone	Sleep pattern/amount

Figure 6.2 Behaviours rated on the Liverpool Infant Distress Score (Horgan *et al.*, 1996)

Score for Facial Expression

0 Eyelids closed and relaxed – no lines, lips slightly apart. No movement of nostril or face.

1 Eyelids remain closed but face slightly screwed up with line around mouth, eyes and over brow. Transient expression and may be repeated often. Baby still asleep but may make mewing noises and sighs with consequent expression.

2 Attentive, receptive expression. Awake and aware and responding to surroundings. Paying interest, no lines on face, slow blinking of eyes. Mouth slowly opening and closing with tongue moving slowly in and out.

3 Eyes partly closed with lines around. Mild furrowing of brow. Face slightly contorted into frown expression. Chin may quiver, gaze may be squinted and brow look 'wary'. May be a transient expression throughout assessment.

4 Moderately furrowed brow. Eyes closed and screwed up tightly causing many lines around eyes. Nostrils sharp and flaring. Lips tightly held, therefore thin line to mouth when crying. Jutting lower lip. May be constant or transient at a ratio of 50:50 with either (3) or (5).

5 Expression held practically all the time without relief. Constant deeply furrowed brow. Very flared nostrils, unnaturally open mouth with tightly held lips. Eyes tightly shut. A grey pallor to face.

Figure 6.3 Score for facial expression

Table 6.3 CRIES pain assessment tool (Krechel and Bilner, 1995)

Parameter	Score		
	0	**1**	**2**
Crying	None	High pitched	Inconsolable
Requires O_2 to keep oxygen saturation > 95 per cent	No	<30 per cent	>30 per cent
Increased vital signs	HR and BP equal to or below preoperative values	HR and BP increased by <20 per cent over preoperative values	HR and BP increased by >20 per cent over preoperative values
Expression	None	Grimace	Grimace/grunt
Sleepless	No	Wakes at frequent intervals	Constantly awake

The problem with any behavioural assessment tool for babies and neonates is of course that it may not be applicable. If the child is

Crying

Facial expression

Verbalisation (both pain and non-pain related)

Movement of the torso

Tactile activity

Leg movements

(McGrath et al., 1985)

Figure 6.4   CHEOPS assessment categories

premature, very ill or receiving sedating drugs, he or she may not demonstrate any behavioural response to pain at all. Pain assessment will then rely on the subjective judgement of the nurse or carer.

A tool devised for children in the immediate postoperative period is the Children's Hospital of Eastern Ontario Pain Scale (CHEOPS) (McGrath et al., 1985). This is based on the categories of pain-related behaviours listed in Figure 6.4. Pain behaviours are scored, the score being said to indicate distress. McGrath (1989) suggests that it is only distress that can be measured as the tool has not been shown to demonstrate pure pain.

The assumption that pain exists in preverbal children can only be just that, an assumption. We all know that many other factors can cause distress behaviour in small children. However, when distress is displayed in the context of a potentially painful condition, whether it is associated with disease, a painful procedure or follows injury or surgery, pain must always be considered to be the principal cause of this distress. Involving parents who have a close and intimate knowledge of how their children respond can make the job very much easier.

When pain may be the source of distress and the response of the infant is observed, analgesic protocols may be developed that help to ensure the timely and adequate management of pain. The following research study by Billmire et al. (1985) demonstrates the benefits of a protocol and also highlights the possibility that small children may actually have a greater need for adequate analgesia than older children.

Protocol development

Billmire *et al.* (1985) studied 2000 children between the ages of 12 months and 12 years who were undergoing a repair of facial lacerations. Using 2–3 µg/kg body weight of fentanyl, good analgesia was achieved and the children's faces were sutured. It was noted, however, that children aged 18–36 months required the full calculated dose of analgesia, while older children usually required less than the calculated dose. It was also noted that a major benefit of good analgesia was that when children returned to have their sutures removed, they were less fearful than children who had not received similar analgesia.

The benefits of a protocol such as the one above might relate to the removal of potential anxieties associated with the administration of analgesia. Other protocols may also be of value, especially when developed for regular routine procedures such as repeated needle-stick procedures in infants, for example taking blood.

Further examples

The process of immunisation frequently involves repeated injections in the first year of an infant's life. Although usually swift, the immediate distress being short lived, 'analgesic' needs are frequently overlooked. A study by Lewindon, *et al.* (1998) reported the benefits of administering 2 ml 75 per cent sucrose by mouth to healthy term infants undergoing needlestick procedures for immunisation. Sucrose may prove a simple, safe and effective means of reducing the distress experienced by infants as the taste has been shown to stimulate endogenous cerebral opioid pathways in a laboratory setting (Kanarek *et al.*, 1991; Zhang *et al.*, 1994).

Time out The previous study illustrates how a simple analgesia protocol can reduce pain and stress.

Can you think of some other non-pharmacological strategies that may be useful to reduce the pain and stress of short painful procedures in the very young child?

How did you get on with the exercise? Many of the traditional non-pharmacological strategies, especially psychological techniques, are applicable only to the fully verbal patient. Strategies such as information-giving or using positive imagery can hardly be applied to the newborn, but there are other therapies that might be of value, especially when used in combination with analgesia:

- *Relieving the problem* – Could the pain possibly be alleviated by overcoming the cause? This may well be the best solution, for example by splinting a painful limb, or inserting a nasogastric tube if abdominal distension might be causing discomfort.
- *Distraction therapy* – If possible, feeding during any procedure that may cause pain can be useful. Giving a baby sucrose can reduce distress; as stated above, it has been suggested that sucrose can stimulate the release of endogenous endorphins.
- *Relaxation therapy* – Gentle touch and massage may well be as beneficial to small children as it is to adults (Beck, 1988). Not only can massage relax and soothe, as a form of cutaneous stimulation, it may also help to close the 'pain gate' referred to in Chapter 1.
- *Comfort strategies* – Keep the baby warm, and eliminate loud noise and bright light. Ensure that examination, nappy changes and turning are done at the same time, rather than constantly disturbing the baby and causing further pain.
- *Cold therapy* – A refrigerant spray, for example, can cool an area prior to inserting a needle.

Much more research is needed, but at least we now have a better understanding of the neurological development of small children. Given that there was virtually no research published before the mid-1980s that focused on children's pain (Jerrett, 1985), the situation is gradually beginning to improve. The basic pharmacological principles are coming under more intense scrutiny. We also have some assessment tools to work with that are based on the observation of facial expression and on behavioural and psychological measures. The education of health care professionals to dispel some long-held myths is still a priority, but at last the issues of pain in children and neonates are becoming a feature of contemporary research. The development of specialised pain assessment tools has been very helpful; it is now essential to get them utilised effectively in practice. Striving to improve our knowledge and involving parents and close relatives can be a positive step towards recognising and treating the pain experienced by some of the most vulnerable patients in our care. For further reading, see the *UK Guidelines and Implementation Guide*, developed by the Royal College of Nursing and the charity Action for Sick Children (1999).

ETHNIC MINORITIES

Since the late 1940s, researchers have been intrigued by the influence that cultural background may have on the experience and expression of pain. We all are aware that people respond quite differently to painful stimuli. Some may become extremely vocal and distressed following what appear to be relatively minor stimuli; other individuals, however, appear unconcerned by what seem to be extremely painful stimuli. A society may value and encourage stoicism, the British 'stiff upper lip' being a good example of how expectations may influence an individual's response. On the other hand, another culture may expect pain to be accompanied by a vigorous verbal and behavioural response.

Melzack and Wall's Gate Control Theory of pain helped to provide a physiological explanation for this variation in pain tolerance and expression. Cultural difference may also substantially influence our response to pain as a result of us modelling our behaviour on how others, similar to us, have behaved. When we experience pain, we draw on this model, our pain behaviour somehow reflecting our cultural background. The research certainly seems to give these theories credence, with fascinating studies of very different reactions to painful encounters that to our Western eyes would seem too terrible to bear.

A child in a large family who is brought up not to fear pain but to accept it as an inevitable part of life may react quite differently from an only child who has been cosseted and experienced a dramatic parental reaction to every small bruise and scratch. In their book *The Challenge of Pain* (1996), Melzack and Wall discuss several cultures and the different ways in which certain people accept pain, often as part of a religious ceremony. Zborowski (1952) was the author of some key work that looked at the response to pain by groups of Irish, Italian and Anglo-American individuals, concluding that definite cultural differences could be predicted. Numerous other studies have been conducted, but the methodology and analysis of findings can be problematic when dealing with an experience as subjective as pain.

Activity

Have you nursed many patients from a cultural background different from your own who were expressing pain in a way you did not expect?

If you have, make a few notes on how they were responding. Discuss these with an experienced colleague.

Have they noted any differences in the way in which certain ethnic minorities respond to pain?

Did these differences make pain assessment more challenging?

It would seem not only that culture and ethnic background influence an individual's response to pain, but that there is also evidence that our own background can influence how we as nurses respond to others in pain. Davitz and Pendelton (1969) and Davitz and Davitz (1985) reported that nurses were influenced not just by cultural differences in patients, but also by their own cultural background, age and social class. Negative stereotyping can sometimes occur when we experience cultural practices or behaviour that differ from those regarded as our own cultural norm.

Childbirth has been studied with a view to delivering equity of care, an issue taken up in *The Patient's Charter* (DoH, 1991). This document states that the health service should set standards that aim for 'respect for privacy, dignity and religious and cultural beliefs and arrangements to ensure everyone, including those with special needs can use the service', but this certainly does not always seem to be the case. A small-scale ethnographic study undertaken by Bowler (1993), which looked at the experience of childbirth in mothers of south-Asian descent, discussed the stereotypical views held by some midwives, which contained four main themes:

149

- difficulty in communication
- the women's lack of compliance with the care available and their abuse of the service
- their tendency to 'make a fuss about nothing'
- their lack of 'normal maternal instinct'.

Women with little English were branded as 'rude and unintelligent', some midwives expressing the view that language difficulties were 'the patients' problem'. From this study, it can clearly be seen that difficulties with health care for ethnic minorities can be experienced because of a lack of understanding of or sensitivity to the effects that background can have on how we deal with pain and stress. Like so many of the challenges that pain may bring to care, there is, when communication is a problem, evidence that nurses may experience negative feelings, may distance themselves from the patient or may limit themselves to giving 'physical' or 'routine' care (Forrest, 1989).

If a culture values stoicism in the face of pain and hardship, adjusting to individuals inclined to respond to pain publicly or vocally can lead to conflict and negative stereotyping, an issue that clearly needs to be addressed. Our cultural background may influence every aspect of our experience of pain from how we react, what treatment we seek and the intensity and duration of the pain we tolerate, to when we report pain, whom we report it to and what type of pain requires attention (Meinhart and McCaffery, 1983). Understanding this cultural influence on pain will prepare us better to cope with a response that is either unexpected or alarming when placed in the context of our own beliefs and culture.

CONCLUSION

The observation of visual or behavioural indicators of pain is only useful when incorporated into a systematic strategy of observation, planning and regular evaluation. Although we lack assessment tools for particularly vulnerable patients, we also lack a culture of regular pain assessment. Regular assessment is vital if we are going to be able effectively to trial a therapy and evaluate its effect. Evaluation is the final and most critical step in managing pain. The evaluation of any strategies can only be based on careful monitoring, and for that one needs a basic observation strategy that enables observed signs of possible pain to be documented and treatments evaluated in light of these documented observations.

For cognitively impaired groups of patients, analgesia may be especially hard to evaluate, and many of the psychological strategies to improve pain relief require a high level of cognitive function, something that will be lacking in this group of patients. The situation is, however, improving and the further reading section will direct you to more in-depth texts.

Where language and culture create barriers to effective pain management, more thought may perhaps need to be given to extending the role of interpreters and encouraging a greater involvement of the family. The inclusion of cultural studies in both pre- and postregistration education will help to raise the awareness of possible problems and conflicts. Preparing health care professionals to deal effectively with potential misunderstandings may ultimately reduce their impact on patient care.

After a break, try the multiple-choice questionnaire below in order to self-assess your learning so far.

Suggested further reading

Bell, M. (1997) Postoperative pain management for the cognitively impaired older adult. *Seminars in Perioperative Nursing*, **6**(1): 37–41.

Carter, B. (ed.) (1994) *Child and Infant Pain. Principles of Nursing Care and Management*, London, Chapman & Hall. (Sections cover neonatal pain memory, cultural influences and infant pain assessment.)

Carter, B. (ed.) (1998) *Perspectives on Pain: Mapping the Territory*, London, Arnold. (Chapter 5, by Bryn Davis, contains a useful discussion of the cultural dimensions of pain.)

Closs, S.J. (1996) Pain and elderly patients: a survey of nurses' knowledge and experiences. *Journal of Advanced Nursing*, **23**: 237–42.

Farrell, M., Katz, B. and Helme, R. (1996) The impact of dementia on the pain experience (review). *Pain*, **67**: 7–15.

Ferrell, B.A. (ed.) (1996) *Clinics in Geriatric Medicine: Pain Management*, Philadelphia, W.B. Saunders.

Hayes, R. (1995) Pain assessment in the elderly. *British Journal of Nursing*, **4**(20): 1199–204.

McKenzie, I.M., Gaukroger, P.B., Ragg, P.G. and Brown, T.C.K. (1997) *Manual of Acute Pain Management in Children*, London, Churchill Livingstone. (An excellent book on acute pain with a special chapter on pain relief in the newborn.)

Parsons, E.P. (1992) Cultural aspects of pain. *Surgical Nurse*, **5**(2): 14–16.

Ranjan, R. (ed.) (1995) *Chronic Pain in Old Age: An Integrated Biospsychosocial Perspective*, Toronto, University of Toronto Press.

Thomas, N.V. (ed.) (1997) *Pain: Its Nature and Management*, London, Baillière Tindall. (Specific chapters deal with the management of children's pain and management strategies for pain in the elderly.)

Walker, J., Akinsanya, J.A., Davis, B. and Marcer, D. (1990) The nursing management of elderly patients with pain in the community: study and recommendations. *Journal of Advanced Nursing*, 15: 1154–61.

Managing Pain in Vulnerable Patients

MULTIPLE-CHOICE QUESTIONNAIRE

1. Historically, pain management in neonates has been neglected. The main reason for this has been:

   a. A lack of reliable and valid pain assessment tools ☐

   b. A belief that neonates do not feel pain ☐

   c. A significant lack of research available to guide practice development ☐

   d. The fact that treatment for pain using opioids was risky and therefore best avoided ☐

2. Which of the following two parameters have been used to assess pain in the neonate?

   a. Crying and reflexes ☐

   b. Crying and appetite ☐

   c. Sleep and physical activity ☐

   d. Vital signs and facial expression ☐

3. Which pain assessment and evaluation tool do you feel could be the most effective for use with the cognitively impaired elderly?

   a. A visual analogue score ☐

   b. A verbal rating ☐

   c. A behavioural rating score ☐

   d. A pain diary ☐

4. When developing an assessment tool based on behaviour, how can individual assessor bias be avoided?

   a. By only having one assessor ☐

   b. By always incorporating an objective measurement, for example pulse or blood pressure ☐

   c. By making sure that everyone is well trained and attends an education session ☐

   d. By ensuring that it possesses explicit criteria for measurement ☐

MULTIPLE-CHOICE QUESTIONNAIRE (cont'd)

5. Effective pain assessment in the brain-injured person depends on:

a. Their chronological age ☐

b. The level of disability resulting from the brain injury ☐

c. The clinical experience of the assessor ☐

d. The evidence of pain-eliciting pathology ☐

6. Whom do you feel would be the most accurate in assessing pain in cognitively impaired patients who cannot communicate verbally?

a. Doctors ☐

b. Nurses ☐

c. Health care assistants ☐

d. Relatives ☐

7. Correctly matching the source of pain with its type, which of the following is correct?

a. Virus infection AND post-herpetic neuralgia ☐

b. Diabetes pain AND intermittent claudication of the legs ☐

c. Musculoskeletal pain AND nerve compression ☐

d. Cancer pain AND joint pain, especially of the large joints ☐

8. Which of the following is a poor indicator of pain that is no longer acute in an adult patient unable to communicate?

a. An alteration in blood pressure ☐

b. Facial expression ☐

c. Altered social interaction ☐

d. A change in posture ☐

9. Osteoarthritis is thought to affect the following percentage of the population:

a. 2 per cent ☐

b. 10 per cent ☐

c. 20 per cent ☐

d. 25 per cent ☐

10. When cognitively impaired patients experience a severe acute injury, when should they receive analgesia?

a. Only when they show obvious signs of distress ☐

b. Whenever they display changes in behaviour or facial expression ☐

c. On a regular basis, based on the duration of action of the drug ☐

d. When they are moved or have some procedure done for them ☐

ANSWERS FOR THE MULTIPLE-CHOICE QUESTIONNAIRE

1.   c. **A significant lack of research available to guide practice development**; until research began to be published, there was little evidence to convince clinicians that practice needed to change. This evidence did not start to emerge until the mid-1980s (Jerrett, 1985). Although the development of reliable and valid pain assessment tools was imperative for the effective management of pain, this was not the main factor involved. For many years, it was a widely held belief that neonates did not have the neural development to feel pain so pain management was not deemed necessary; this has only recently been disproved. Treatment for pain in neonates using opioids was risky and therefore best avoided, although this was a factor that discouraged clinicians from prescribing and administering opioids; again, however, it was not the main reason.

2.   d. **Vital signs and facial expression;** both have been used in the CRIES scale of Krechel and Bilner (1995). Crying and vital signs have been used in assessment parameters, but reflexes have not. Neither has appetite, which although it might be affected by pain, is not a reliable measure. Sleep has been used, as have leg movements (McGrath et al. 1985) but not 'physical activity', the latter being difficult to measure objectively.

3.   c. **A verbal rating;** it appears that even in the severely cognitively impaired patient, the ability to provide some sort of verbal rating for pain can be used. Where speech is non-existent, a behavioural rating score is the first choice but it does appear that we often tend to overlook a patient's ability to communicate their pain even when, in other areas, communication is severely hampered. It is unlikely that a visual analogue score could be used, but a pain diary kept by relatives or carers might be of value.

4.   d. **By ensuring that it possesses explicit criteria for measurement;** clear criteria will reduce the chance of assessor bias and improve the reliability of the scale, as, for example, in the LIDS scale (Horgan et al., 1996). Only having one assessor might reduce the chance of error between assessors, but it is not practical and the assessor would still need to know what to look for to rate the pain. Although it might be useful to incorporate an objective measurement, for example pulse or blood pressure, it is important that scales do not rely solely on one dimension of expression; again, this would not be practical. Making sure that everyone is well trained and attends an education session is important and would help, but it is not the prime answer as people could still make their own interpretations.

5.   b. **The level of disability resulting from the brain injury;** this is critical in terms of assessing the patient's pain. Understanding how much cognitive impairment he or she has will influence the choice of assessment tool and the contribution that the patient can make. For the assessment of pain, chronological age will not be a key factor, but cognitive age and ability will be. The clinical experience of the assessor will not necessarily be relevant as there will be many situations in which the main carer rather than the nurse will assess the pain. The evidence of pain-eliciting pathology is important in the context of the pain experience but does not relate explicitly to the assessment of pain.

6.   d. **Relatives** would appear to be better than all health care professionals at assessing pain in patients who cannot communicate. Parents with severely brain-injured

children seem especially able to pick up signals of pain and discomfort that to an outsider are extremely subtle and difficult to identify.

7. a. **Virus infection AND post-herpetic neuralgia** is correct. Viruses of the herpes family can lie dormant in nerves, shingles being an example of post-herpetic neuralgia. Diabetes pain elicits peripheral neuropathy. Musculoskeletal problems such as osteoporosis cause fractures and contractures. Cancer pain elicits a range of pain types but not specifically joint pain in larger joints; the latter would be the typical pain of arthritis.

8. a. **An alteration in blood pressure** is physiologically demanding, and once pain is no longer acute, the body adapts. Chronic pain can often elicit no obvious pathological changes. Observations of facial expression, altered social interaction and change in posture have all been used to assess pain.

9. b. **10 per cent;** it is thought that 10 per cent of the population suffers from osteoarthritis, although this is primarily associated with ageing.

10. c. **On a regular basis, based on the duration of action of the drug,** would seem to be the most humane method, combined with regular assessment and evaluation to ensure that the medication is working, is still needed and is not producing side-effects. This will obviously require a great deal of skill, but given that all the evidence, especially surrounding the elderly and cognitively impaired, indicates that we have managed pain very badly in the past, pre-empting any obvious signs of pain for a few days seems sensible. Unfortunately, the effective observation of behavioural signs for assessment purposes is only just being developed.

7 Nursing patients with challenging pain

LEARNING OUTCOMES

On completion of this chapter the student will be able to:

■ Identify two groups of clients for whom pain management will be particularly challenging

■ Discuss factors that contribute to pain being inadequately or inappropriately managed for these people

■ Critically analyse the challenging aspects related to pain management for an individual you have cared for

■ Evaluate strategies that might lead to improved pain relief for the individual selected in the previous learning outcome

INDICATIVE READING

Atkinson, J.H., Slater, M.A., Patterson, T.L., Grant, I. and Garfin, S.R. (1988) Depressed mood in chronic low back pain: relationship with stressful life events. *Pain*, **35**: 47–55.

Cromey, S. (1998) The pain of withdrawing from illicit heroin use. In Carter, B. (ed.) *Perspective on Pain: Mapping the Territory*, London, Arnold, p. 306.

Dworkin, R.H., Handlin, D.S., Richlin, D.M., Brand, L. and Vannucci, C. (1985) Unravelling the effects of compensation, litigation, and employment on treatment response in chronic pain. *Pain*, **23**: 49–59.

Judkins, K. (1998) Pain management in the burned patient. *Pain Reviews*, **5**: 133–46.

Keefe, K.J., Wilkins, R.H., Cook, W.A., Crisson, J.E. and Muhlbaier, J.H. (1986) Depression, pain and pain behaviour. *Journal of Consulting and Clinical Psychology*, **54**: 665–9.

McCaffery, M. and Vourakis, C. (1992) Assessment and relief of pain in chemically dependent patients. *Orthopaedic Nursing*, **11**(2): 13–27.

Seddon, R. and Savage, M.D. (1993) Addiction in the treatment of pain: significance, recognition and management. *Journal of Pain and Symptom Management*, **8**(5): 265–77.

Skevington, S. (1995) *Psychology of Pain*, Chichester, John Wiley & Sons.

Thomas, V.J. and Westerdale, N. (1997) Sickle cell disease. *Nursing Standard*, **11**(25): 40–7.

Tyrer, S. (ed.) (1992) *Psychology, Psychiatry and Chronic Pain*, (see Chapters 3–6). Oxford, Butterworth-Heinemann.

BACKGROUND

Although pain is an individual and unique experience, previous chapters on the management of acute and chronic pain have considered the 'normal' pattern of events. This chapter captures a range of pain experiences that have received relatively scant attention in the literature but, as in the vulnerable patient, often afford a great challenge to clinicians. While we may not offer the answers here, we hope to raise your awareness, stimulate a dialogue and provide reference material, relevant articles and supportive ideas.

The need for a chapter such as this stems from a growing demand from the public for health care to define a cause for a disorder, especially a painful one, treat the cause and solve the problem. Unfortunately, for many in society, the symptom of pain is not so straightforward, but success in other spheres of health care fuels the demand to cure all ills. We now live in a society that has high expectations of what health care can deliver, and those in pain are no longer prepared to suffer in silence. However, when we are faced with pain that challenges our ability to relieve it, or even in some cases understand it, the encounter can be frustrating and unsatisfactory for staff and patients alike. The term 'heart-sink' sometimes springs to mind when one is left to confront the patient with mountainous notes for whom no therapy so far has appeared to offer any control of pain or relief of suffering.

We shall first consider the care of patients with particularly challenging pain that can occur as a result of major tissue damage or disease, following burns or spinal injuries. Next, we will look at people with sickle-cell disease, who can experience intense, life-threatening pain crises, which are often inadequately unrelieved. Mood disorders, covered after this, can be powerful in altering our perception of pain, and for some patients their pain may be associated with secondary gain. This may not be consciously sought but can be significant in terms of the part it can play in recovery. The development of intractable, unrelieved pain can also have life-changing consequences. Then comes substance abuse, a huge social issue, the management of pain with these people requiring a clear understanding of the need to reduce their pain effectively when they enter the health care system. Each section of the chapter outlines the issues and makes suggestions on strategies to improve pain management. It is assumed that the assessment of pain is a necessary prerequisite prior to the selection of any interventions, and you may at some time wish to refer back to Chapter 2.

Activity

Go to the library and look up in the index of several contemporary pain textbooks the following topic areas:

- substance abuse

- burns

- spinal injuries

- intractable pain

How many books actually contained text related to these problems?

It is likely that very few of these issues appeared in a textbook or, if they did, they were mentioned in passing. Another way of considering the scope of a topic is to look at the contents page of a book and work out how many pages are actually dedicated to the topic you are interested in and what percentage of the book they form.

It is helpful to consider how the topics we are to explore fit within the multidimensional framework of pain. The two main categories of pain can be defined by their cause: is the pain based on a pathophysiological disorder or a psychological disorder driven by disordered perception and behaviour? Figure 7.1 is rather simplistic as, in reality, pain is a complex mixture of both categories. It is helpful to view pain as a continuum with physical causes at one end and psychosocial influence at the other. Figure 7.1 illustrates the importance of consid-

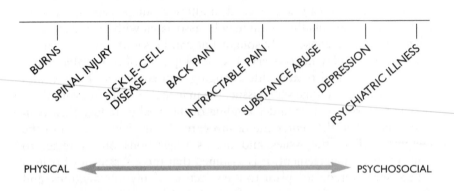

Figure 7.1   Physical and psychological influences on pain

ering the physical influences on all the conditions given and how these influences may move up and down a continuum. It might also be useful here to refer to Chapter 1.

PAIN FOLLOWING A SERIOUS BURN

People who have experienced burns have several needs, all of which impact on their experience of pain. Pain management is an essential and an integral part of their nursing care, and will increasingly become part of the non-specialist nursing role as burns treatment centres are reduced in number (Atkinson, 1998), yet pain has a poor record of being managed effectively (Ulmer, 1998). This section will consider why people who have been burnt have special needs, as well as other key aspects of their pain management.

Special needs

The pain of a burn is known to us all. We have all at one time or another been unfortunate enough to catch our hand on a cooker, in a fire, in steam or with boiling water. It used to be assumed that the larger the area of burn, the greater the pain, and the deeper the burn, the less pain because of the nerve endings being destroyed within the deeper tissue damage. In practice, most deep burn areas are intermingled with damage to superficial elements, and pain is usually a definite sequela. A burn will also damage tissue, sometimes irreparably, resulting in long-term disfigurement and anguish from these scars. The emotional turmoil can contribute significantly to the experience of pain.

Time out   Have you ever had a serious burn, or do you know someone who has experienced one?

What was the pain like?

Did the pain change over time?

Was pain related to any particular activity?

It was likely that the pain was initially intense and sharp but that the administration of cold (usually running) water then reduced the pain sensation. Later, a deep throbbing pain might have emerged, along with anxiety about the consequences of the burn and how it would heal. Day-to-day background discomfort is there most of the time, and it may be painful to move the affected limb. It should be remembered that many burns involve children, and it has already been described how their pain is often neglected and presents the practitioner with additional challenges related to assessment (see Chapter 6).

Changing the dressing

Time out   When you take a sticking plaster off, how do you feel?
Imagine that the sticking plaster has stuck to your burn or cut, and a friend comes along and offers to help to rip the tape off.
What do you say?

It is likely that the initial pain you experience when you come to take the plaster off makes you anxious about the pain you predict you will feel. If a friend offers to remove it for you, you will probably decline (most kindly of course) as you will prefer to have control of this pain-eliciting activity yourself.

In clinical situations, we often take this control away from patients by not allowing them to participate in their dressing changes. Research with burns patients has demonstrated that by allowing them to participate in their own dressing changes, they experience significantly less pain (Sutherland, 1996). It has also been shown that reducing the number of times the dressing is changed can reduce the pain associated with dressing change. Sheridan *et al.* (1997) undertook a research study with 50 burned children and found that a once-daily change resulted in no significant alteration in infection morbidity compared with twice-daily changing.

Madjar (1998) has written an excellent book on her own research, which explores the *lived experience* of pain inflicted in the context of medically prescribed treatment. Based on interviews with burns patients and those receiving chemotherapy, she explores the infliction of pain from both the patient's and nurse's perspective. Without an understanding of inflicted pain, nurses are ill prepared to reduce the incidence or prevalence of such pain or manage their own feelings of stress when they have to inflict pain. It is a thought-provoking book that helps us understand rather than feel guilty.

Psychosocial interventions

The devastating nature of a burn increases the psychological and physiological responses of the person involved. Although the pain of burns can be treated by analgesic interventions, it is the inclusion of psychological strategies that enhance the effectiveness of pain management. See Judkins (1998) for an excellent résumé of analgesic interventions.

Activity

If you were caring for someone with a burn, what strategies would you utilise to complement the analgesia they might be taking?

Would there be any special considerations for the selection of these?

Psychological methods, which are useful, include cognitive and behavioural interventions. If the patient is unable to move easily, the use of a video or music for distraction could be helpful. Think about where the dressing changes take place. If the unit has a specific 'room', what could be done to make this a pleasant environment that might take someone's mind off the pain? If the walls are plain, how about inviting an artist in to create some murals? This could be done in partnership with the patients as they might have some ideas too. Can you play music or have the TV available? Don't forget the ceiling – a mobile or pictures can be more interesting than a blank space.

Nowadays, there are also catalogues available that contain many items of distraction therapy from equipment, toys and special interactive books, to bubble tubes and so on, from which everyone can benefit. Most of these are targeted at children and those with learning difficulties, either to stimulate their environment or to distract attention away from something that is potentially unpleasant.

From personal experience, it can be very useful to keep interactive, distracting toys and therapies in a special box, to be used only when an inflicted pain of short duration is unavoidable. For children, the use of these distracting toys can have a 'knock-on' benefit that is not just confined to the child. Interactive toys and books can distract and calm an anxious parent who may be subconsciously transmitting his or her fear and apprehension to the child. For adults and children alike, it can be worthwhile using visually distracting strategies such as lava lamps and fibreoptic lamps that constantly change colour, as well as equipment that will project all sorts of colours, lights and images onto the walls and ceilings. Behavioural interventions such as relaxation have also been effective (Judkins, 1998). Psychosocial interventions are discussed in further detail by Davis and Sheely-Adolphson (1997).

Activity

Next time you have to carry out an activity on a patient that might cause some discomfort, try using some form of distraction. For example, if the procedure is to be undertaken on a child, try getting somebody to read from a large book that obscures the child's view of what you are doing. If possible, get the child to suck on a boiled sweet at the same time. Remember that sucrose on a dummy sucked by a baby can reduce the crying time of babies having a needle stick (Lewindon et al., 1998).

PAIN IN THE PATIENT WITH A SPINAL INJURY

The effective management of pain continues to be a significant problem in people with spinal cord injuries, but there is little agreement on the nature of pain and the definitions of different types of pain following such trauma (Siddall et al., 1997).

Activity

Why do you think this might be, and what implications could this have for people with spinal cord injuries?

A quick review of textbooks on spinal injuries reveals an alarming absence of the discussion of pain. This might erroneously lead the reader to believe that pain is not a problem for these people, or that its management is straightforward and does not warrant special consideration. This is, in reality, far from the truth. One study found that 64 per cent of 353 patients experienced pain following spinal injury (Levi *et al.*, 1995). The early detection and management of pain is essential. Bowsher (1999) has written an excellent paper on the importance of discerning between central pain caused by nociceptive (tissue damage) and neurogenic (pathological changes in the nervous system) pain in the person with spinal cord injury. The importance of the distinction between the two is essential as their treatment is completely different.

Research summary

The distinction is made between two different pathophysiological varieties of pain in the person with a spinal cord injury: pain resulting from tissue damage (which responds to opioids) and neuropathic pain (which rarely does). Neuropathic pain is complex because it results from pathological changes in the nervous system, which can be central or peripheral. Interventions aimed at interfering with traditional pain pathways, for example opioids, may be ineffective. Neuropathic pain, which involves damage to the central nervous system, is often called central pain. Many patients with neuropathic pain complain of burning or icy pain, some have allodynia (pain elicited by light touch) and the onset of this pain often occurs much later. The treatment of neuropathic pain has relied on drugs such as antidepressants (for example, amitriptyline) that inhibit central mechanisms. Their antidepressant action appears to be separate from their analgesic action. Treatment profiles suggest that the earlier these patients are treated, the better the outcome, and where the likelihood of central pain is very high, as with spinal cord injury, their pre-emptive use is recommended. For further information, see Bowsher (1999).

Time out Why is it so important that pain in the person with a spinal injury is managed effectively?

Several reasons emerge to treat pain in spinal injury patients effectively. Survivors are often grappling with multiple injuries and may have been fortunate to have escaped death. This life-changing circumstance is accompanied by a turmoil of emotions. The advent of pain in an area of their body that they can no longer feel, or use as they previously did, can cause anxiety and possibly hope (that this signals healing). It may also be difficult to understand as the physiology is complex, and if health care professionals dismiss their pain, sufferers may feel isolated, vulnerable and angry. The medical treatment of spinal cord injuries has considerably increased life expectancy, and the experience of living with chronic pain should not be the reward for survival.

Quality of life is a critical factor for the survivor of an injury. Wagner Anke *et al.* (1995) found that reduced quality of life and psychological distress was more prevalent in patients with pain than in those without pain. Pain will obviously impair an individual's ability to cope with the severe impairment of these devastating injuries, and its effective management should, from the beginning, be integral to the plan of care for these people.

PAIN IN PATIENTS WITH SICKLE-CELL DISEASE

Sickle-cell disease is the result of a group of genetic blood disorders characterised by a gene mutation that leads to the production of an abnormal haemoglobin (HbS). The shape of this haemoglobin is different because of its 'sickle' shape, which can lead to clumping of the cells during a 'crisis', causing extreme pain as they block the fine capillaries. It is estimated that 129 babies are born each year with the disease (Modell and Anionwu, 1996). An excellent discussion of pathophysiology, strategies for management and psychological considerations can be found in Thomas (1998).

Activity

Find out which group of patients are usually affected by this disease.

In your community, how are the health needs of these people addressed?

This chronic disease can profoundly affect both sufferers and their families. They live with the uncertainty of the disease and the fear of a 'painful crisis', which can cause not only severe pain and illness, but possibly also death. Because of the prevalence of the disease within a culture that is often different from that of most health care professionals, these people sometimes feel neglected and disbelieved, their needs going unmet. In particular, the attitude of the health care professional can profoundly influence the effectiveness of pain management.

Living with a chronic and potentially life-threatening disease can affect the psychological well-being of these people, an issue that is highlighted in an excellent paper by Thomas *et al.* (1998).

Research summary

The advent of a painful crisis is the most common symptom of this disease and is responsible for the second greatest number of admissions to hospital in London, patients remaining in hospital for an average of 7 days. The management of pain has been found to be less than adequate, resulting in stress and anxiety for individuals and their families. Evidence from the United States suggests that cognitive-behavioural therapy (CBT) is successful when combined with other pain management strategies, reduced psychological distress and fewer hospital admissions being the main outcomes. Thomas *et al.* (1998) provide a particularly useful discussion of CBT in sickle-cell disease.

Activity

After reading the article by Thomas *et al.* (1998), cited above, make notes for the following questions:

- Why might people with sickle-cell disease be at risk of developing psychological problems?

- What is the aim of CBT?

- How can CBT be used with people who have sickle-cell disease?

Sickle-cell disease affects individuals from the moment they are born. Thomas and Westerdale (1997) review the nursing management of these patients and reflect on the impact of the disease at various points in the development of the child from infancy through to early adulthood. With survival being more precarious in the first 5 years of life and again at around 20–24 years of age, life expectancy is still only around 40 years. For those people carrying the HbS, which causes the sickle-cell shape in red blood cells, the disease usually manifests itself before the age of 6. The highest mortality occurs in this age group, usually as a result of infection, which precipitates a crisis.

Time out   Imagine what it might be like to have this disease.
How might your early experiences of a painful crisis affect you later in life?

Our experience of pain is affected by many variables, previous experience being just one of them. If you have been repeatedly admitted to hospital and your pain has not been managed effectively, you will probably feel very anxious when you have to return. This anxiety, pain and frustration will probably affect the way in which you behave towards the hospital staff. You may feel alienated and misunderstood or disbelieved. Schechter (1985) suggests that sickle-cell disease is exacerbated by prejudice as it usually affects black and poor people, whereas health care providers are usually white and middle class (see Chapter 6).

To ensure that a painful crisis is managed effectively, it is essential that health care professionals can assess pain accurately and establish a real belief in a patient's pain. The management of sickle-cell pain can be a helpful model for other types of chronic pain (Gorman, 1999).

In an insightful paper, Alleyne and Thomas (1994) interviewed 10 patients who suffered from sickle-cell disease about their care. All 10 expressed dissatisfaction with the management of their pain crises. Some of the difficulties, for example not being believed and having to wait for analgesia, are familiar problems for other groups of patients too.

MOOD DISORDER AND PAIN

In some cases, psychological disorder may contribute to pain perception. However, this can be used as an excuse by health care professionals to explain pain that is confounding a diagnosis or organic explanation. As we begin very gradually to unravel some of the intricacies of pain, psychology and psychiatry it is already possible to identify several psychiatric disorders that may be involved in pain perception (Merskey and Chandarana, 1992):

- anxiety
- depression
- hypochondriasis
- somatisation disorder
- Munchausen syndrome.

Anxiety

A relationship between anxiety and acute pain has been well established. Walsh (1993) studied pain and anxiety in an accident and emergency (A&E) department and reported the value of keeping patients informed. Anxiety may result in increased muscle tension that can ultimately lead to pain and fatigue. For further information read Walding (1991), and see also Chapter 3.

Depression

Experiencing chronic pain would make anybody depressed, but in some instances it is difficult to establish exactly which came first: depression, leading an individual to become predisposed to pain, or pain causing the individual to become depressed about his or her situation. The association between pain and depression is not well understood, although its existence is well documented (Skevington, 1995). It has been suggested that some chronic pain patients may overestimate the intensity of past painful episodes because the mood associated with their current pain is similar to the mood they experienced when they first had the pain. Like so many of the psychosocial factors surrounding pain, more research is needed to establish possible links.

Hypochondriasis

This condition has been described as an overawareness of bodily sensation leading to an apprehension of disease and phobic concern.

It is suggested that this term is overused and obsolete, too often being used by clinicians when pain proves difficult to explain.

Somatisation disorder

'Somatic pain' is a term normally used to describe pain in cutaneous and deeper tissues such as bone, ligaments and muscle. 'Somatisation disorder', however, is a term used to describe pain that is said to arise in late adolescence or the early twenties in patients who present with a history of multiple complaints, often occurring in clusters, for which no sufficient physical cause can be found (Tyler, 1992). The term seems to be used these days to describe what in the past was claimed to be hypochondriasis. Assessment for atypical masked depression should be included in the differential diagnosis in elderly patients with somatic complaints and multidisciplinary management is recommended, with the inclusion of a psychiatrist. Maue (1986) contains further information on this subject.

Munchausen syndrome

This is a very complex psychological disorder that is only just beginning to be studied and understood. The reader is referred to Kleinman (1988) for an exposition of this complex condition, and to Parnell and Day (1998) for literature that may throw some light on the origins of Muchausen syndrome within families.

case history

Mary has been admitted to the female surgical ward with low abdominal pain, increasing in intensity to 8/10 over the 24 hours prior to her admission. Mary is 42 years old and lives with her husband and only child, John, in a small town 100 miles away – they had been staying with her sister locally when her pain started. Over the next 48 hours numerous investigations were carried out, results all being negative. Although kept nil by mouth in case of surgery and using a patient-controlled analgesia pump for pain relief, Mary seemed content with the situation. It was decided that a decision would be made on the Wednesday doctors' round when Professor Richards was available. In the interim 2 days, a large set of notes from her local hospital arrived. The surgical notes catalogued a series of similar painful episodes over the past 10 years, which had resulted in numerous surgical investigations. All had drawn a blank as nothing abnormal could be found.

During the Wednesday round, Professor Richards sat down with Mary and her husband and explained as gently as he could that surgery was unlikely to help her pain and that he was not prepared to operate. This news was met with extreme anger and tears from Mary, but this gradually gave way to a different emotion. As Professor Richard's explained that he would not operate because it would not get rid of her pain, he felt he wanted to give her a real chance of getting better and would refer her to someone who would help her with her pain and the havoc it was wreaking with her life. A referral was made to a clinical psychologist, and although our expectations were that Mary would be angry, she was not. That evening she seemed happier and her pain had diminished. Someone had confronted her and realised that she was very unhappy. Recognising this and being strong enough to talk openly about this with her meant that she had the prospect of a new start.

Summary

Disordered thought, perception and behaviour are a new field of study for the pain specialist, and, as stated previously, there is always a danger that when pain cannot be explained easily by the presence of obvious pathological factors, it will automatically be dismissed as being psychological in origin. As we start to understand the complex neurophysiology of pain, there is a risk in thinking that we may have the answers. So often, it would appear an obscure mechanical or pathological source of pain, previously undetected, may be found to explain some pain, but patients have had to deal with the frustration of having their pain 'labelled' as psychological. For chronic pain, an endless search for a definite diagnosis or physical cause can lead to years of frustration, anger and pain. Modern technology does not always have the answers, so it is better to focus on helping someone to live with their pain through effective coping strategies than to search fruitlessly to find out 'why'. When the cause cannot be treated, helping sufferers live with and come to terms with their pain must always be the goal.

SUBSTANCE ABUSE

Pain experienced by patients with a history of substance abuse

There are few clinical situations more challenging, frustrating or stressful than the management of acute or chronic pain in patients known or suspected to be abusers [of chemicals]. (Payne, 1989, p. 46)

How true this statement is to anyone who has ever managed the care of a patient in pain with a history of opioid use for recreation rather than pain relief. In the past, society has tended to just blame patients for their own inadequacies (Stimmel, 1989), but as we are coming to understand more about the dual problems of relieving pain and the complexities of addiction, we are faced with a need to know more about the management of these complicated and challenging patients.

Part of Chapter 1 endeavoured to clarify some of the misconceptions surrounding the terminology associated with substance abuse. To recap we will use the following definitions:

- *Substance abuse* and *addiction* are described as being one and the same, although 'addiction' can cover other areas such as food. In this instance, the terms apply to psychological dependence that is characterised by a compulsive use of drugs for non-medical reasons, a loss of control over the circumstances of drug use, continued use despite adverse consequences, frequent relapses after periods of abstinence and the inability voluntarily to decrease use (World Health Organization, 1986; American Psychiatric Association, 1987; American Pain Society, 1989).

- *Physical dependence* occurs when a patient manifests symptoms of withdrawal when a drug is suddenly stopped – **it is a sign not that a patient is addicted but merely that the patient's body has become dependent on a substance,** often one that mimics an endogenous substance. The sudden withdrawal of this substance can lead to unpleasant side-effects while the body tries to adjust. Although withdrawal symptoms – or 'cold turkey' as it is referred to among addicts and lay people – is often associated with 'drug addiction', non-addicted patients may exhibit the same symptoms. For these patients, the symptoms can always be avoided if the drugs are withdrawn slowly rather than suddenly halted over night.

- *Tolerance* is defined as the need to administer larger doses of a drug in order to obtain the same effect. It usually occurs after repeated doses of opioid-based drugs. Again, it is not a sign of addiction but one of the body becoming 'used' to a drug. In the case of cancer patients, it can often signal an increase in pathology, or disease progression.

Time out   How often in your clinical area do you hear staff and patients voice concerns regarding addiction?
Are their concerns justified? How many patients have a real addiction?

If you have looked after someone with addiction who has pain, was
their pain recognised and adequately controlled?

It is quite probable that these patients did not have their pain properly
recognised and assessed. Have you ever seen 'avoid opioids' written on
the drug charts of patients admitted to hospital with multiple trauma
who happen to be heroin addicts? This strategy indicates that the
patient's pain has not been controlled, and they are left to suffer withdrawal symptoms that cause additional pain and distress. When painful
trauma or disease is present, it is not the time to make judgements or
attempt to get a patient 'off heroin'. In fact, additional opioids will be
necessary, often in very large quantities to overcome tolerance.

Withdrawal is unpleasant and can so easily be avoided provided that
opioids are not stopped rapidly. The symptoms are easy to identify:

- hypertension
- tachycardia
- abdominal pain
- muscle aches
- yawning
- diarrhoea
- rhinorrhea
- lacrimation
- vomiting and diarrhoea
- goosepimples.

The pain of withdrawing from heroin is explored by Cromey, (1998).
Cromey's chapter covers self-detoxification, substitute opioid prescribing and a variety of issues associated with the process. Drawing
on a wealth of research, the only criticism would be the lack of personal narratives, or a patient perspective would have complemented
the text superbly.

Managing pain control in the opioid-abusing patient

You should set realistic goals, stating that although you will endeavour to control the pain as effectively as possible, you may have to
explain to the patient that, because of acquired tolerance, the control
of his or her pain will be more difficult to achieve. These patients

often accept this and in fact expect this to be the case. They can often be disarmingly grateful that anybody is taking the time and effort to recognise and try to alleviate their pain. Many will have had poor past experiences of health care facilities. The very nature of their lifestyle means that they have often experienced pain in the past, as well as being prone to trauma, infection, abscess formation and general ill-health. It might have been their experience on previous hospital admissions to have their pain ignored, their addiction being seen as their own fault.

We cannot underestimate the frustration and negative feelings that many health care professionals experience when having to nurse profoundly ill patients on a busy ward whose condition is a result of self-abuse such as opioid or alcohol addiction. It is all too easy to be judgmental, but we often have no insight into the sort of background that many of these people have endured. Sometimes all they have known is a life on the street; they may present as personally neglected, abusive and difficult. That is, however, probably the only life they know, often coming from an environment that is harsh and dangerous. The only language they are familiar with is abusive and crude. Attempting to manage such patients' pain can, however, offer great reward. Patience and collaboration will frequently lead to the development of a therapeutic relationship that does not have to be negative for staff. We would not presume that the development of this therapeutic relationship is going to be easy; it has to be one of negotiation and teamwork.

The assessment of pain will present special challenges. Although pain rating methods are always subjective, subjectivity is even more apparent in the patient with a history of opioid abuse. A very high pain score will almost always be the norm, but assessment is still necessary for a long-term comparison to evaluate different treatments. Differentiating between a high pain score and drug-seeking pain behaviour can sometimes prove impossible. While a patient is receiving active treatment in hospital is neither the time nor the place to disbelieve or question high pain scores. Nobody likes to be duped by a patient, but as there is no way of verifying patient reports of severe pain, we have no real alternative but to accept what they say.

While patients are in hospital, we have a duty to recognise their pain and do our best to alleviate it, even though in some instances we may suspect that we are being used to fuel a habit. However, denying adequate treatment usually means that the patient will self-discharge or get his or her friends to bring in supplies. This can be dangerous if you do not know how much, or with what, patients are topping up their analgesia. There is also the dilemma of what to do if you suspect that a patient has a locker full of street heroin. Do you breach trust and search the locker, call the police, confront the patient? It is surely much better to foster an open and honest relationship from the start and work collaboratively with the patient; remember too that they will probably know far more about most of these drugs than you do.

case history

Jane is a 21-year-old who has been working for 6 years as a prostitute to fuel a heroin addiction she has had since a boyfriend introduced her to the drug when she was 15. In a desperate bid to end her life, or more probably in a desperate plea for help, she has taken an overdose of sleeping tablets and jumped out of a second-storey window, landing on the grass below. She is unconscious when her friends find her 3 hours later. They think that she was has just had a 'bad trip' and drag her upstairs to bed. The following morning, Jane is conscious and tells her friends she has a terrible pain in her heels, ankles and knees, and that her back hurts. The pain is so bad that she begs her friends to give her a shot of heroin before calling the ambulance. When the ambulance men arrive, they are unsure of what has happened or of the extent of Jane's injuries. She is difficult to rouse, but when she is finally roused, she is abusive and unco-operative.

Jane is taken to the A&E department of her local hospital with a history obtained from her friends that she has taken a drug, has had a bad trip and has fallen over. It is almost impossible to obtain a history from Jane, but the department staff suspect that Jane has been a substance abuser for some time as she has needle marks up both her arms. As a result, she needs a central line in her neck in order for them to obtain intravenous access. Because Jane is so difficult to obtain a history from and her friends have been unable to help, she is given some naloxone to reverse the heroin. She becomes almost impossible to manage, but numerous X-rays enable the A&E staff to confirm that Jane has multiple fractures of her legs, a fracture of her pelvis and a non-displaced fracture of her lower spine.

Although Jane is given some additional opioid pain relief once the naloxone has worn off, the amount is not sufficient to counteract the symptoms of opioid withdrawal that develop quite rapidly. For the next 36 hours, over a weekend, Jane receives totally inadequate analgesia. Threatening to discharge herself from hospital, she is finally seen by the acute pain team in an extremely distressed state. Her pain is described as unbearable, and she is in acute withdrawal.

This case history may seem extreme, but in the authors' experience, it is not that uncommon.

Activity

If you get the opportunity to talk to a patient with a history of opioid abuse, ask them how they would like to have pain managed while they are in hospital.

Many have such bad previous experiences that they are delighted when somebody takes the trouble to obtain information from their perspective.

Key points for effective care of patients with opioid dependency

- If you suspect that a patient may be a drug abuser, try to confirm this as early as possible. Many will be quite honest and open about their addiction, especially if they know that you are trying to control their pain.

- Make sure you contact people with specialist knowledge; your acute pain team, pharmacist, local drug and alcohol clinic, palliative care teams may be able to help.

- Ensure that only one person is responsible for prescribing medication in order to avoid multiple changes and the prescription of incompatible drugs, for example a partial agonist or agonist/antagonist, as this could lead to withdrawal symptoms.

- Use patient-controlled analgesia where practical and possible, remembering that the bolus dose often has to be at least twice or even three times the normal dose.

- Ensure that the patient receives sufficient opioids to control withdrawal and provide pain relief; the doses often have to be very high. Try to establish how much opioid the patient takes on a daily basis, but remember that this will only be a rough guide as street drugs can vary considerably in quality and strength, and some patients will be quite creative for fear that you will underestimate their need. Unfortunately, heroin has in the past few years become cheaper and easier to obtain so patients can often tolerate extremely high doses.

- Where possible, use combination therapy, that is, opioids, non-steroidal anti-inflamatory drugs (NSAIDS), local anaesthetics, adjuvants and non-pharmacological strategies.

● Collaborate with patients, obtaining their trust and setting realistic goals.

INTRACTABLE PAIN AND SECONDARY GAIN

'Intractable' is a term that is often used when, despite everyone's best efforts, a patient's pain remains stubbornly resistant to any sort of influence, therapy or cure. The term 'secondary gain' has been used to describe the possible influence that practical, financial or emotional advantage may have on pain becoming intractable. In instances where a person may gain some advantage from his or her pain, breaking the cycle of pain and pain behaviour can become extremely difficult.

These patients are not malingering, which is described as lying about the existence of pain, and is said to be quite rare (McCaffery and Beebe, 1994). What appears to happen is that an initial injury, which may have been very painful at the time, results in ongoing pain way beyond the time at which acute pain resulting from the injury would have been expected to subside. The pain is very real but could be far more linked to feelings of distress, poor coping strategies, loss of self-esteem and social isolation than many of us might previously have realised. All chronic pain has a psychosocial dimension, but we perhaps currently lack sufficient understanding and skill to be able to unravel the complex interplay between the influence of the body and the mind.

Activity

Do you know a friend, relative or patient who suffers from intractable pain with little, or seemingly insignificant, pathology, but whose pain causes them a great deal of suffering and distress?

Now make a short list of factors that may inhibit strategies to improve how such individuals cope with their pain. Could subtle factors be contributing to the fact that they have not come to terms with their pain and adapted their lives to it? What enables some individuals to live with pain but still enjoy quality of life while others become deeply unhappy, socially isolated and totally overwhelmed? Consider the following:

● workers' compensation
● outstanding litigation
● disability allowance
● attention from health care professionals
● attention from friends and family
● sanctioned avoidance of stress at work
● sanctioned avoidance of domestic role
● reduced responsibility
● loss of feelings of control.

Research is only just beginning to emerge that attempts to describe chronic pain and suffering, influenced not only by our mood, culture and background, but also by a constellation of other factors. When these factors start to interplay adversely, the scene is set for a downwards spiral into pain, immobility and misery.

Dissatisfaction with health care professionals may develop as multiple encounters fail to be effective. This inevitably leads to tension, anger, conflict and possibly hostility. Without a proper explanation for their continuing pain, individuals become increasingly inactive as they associate 'undiagnosed' pain with further damage. They often increase their analgesic drug use, which has a further negative effect on mood and activity. Inactivity leads to joints becoming stiff and painful, scar tissue may contract and muscles waste, and exhaustion and fatigue take over. Patients withdraw from activities and social interactions that used to give them pleasure, focusing more and more on their pain. Dependency sets in, and resentment may spread. When illness behaviour eventually fails to elicit a benevolent response, conflict extends further to friends and family.

Social Policy

It could be argued that we now live within a social infrastructure that may be seen to support dependency rather than the positive strategies that encourage sufferers to return to as normal a life as possible. It is worthwhile considering the vast amount of money, which increases year on year, being paid in disability allowance compared with the tiny fraction of the Chancellor's coffers that is spent on chronic pain clinics, rehabilitation facilities, back schools that teach back pain sufferers to manage life following a back injury, clinical psychologists and psychological therapists who may be able to alter adverse pain behaviour. Consider also the fact that we now have aggressive health and safety policies within the workplace, with a steep decline in the number of heavy and hazardous industries such as coal mining. Between 1986 and 1992, however, the figure for disability benefit being paid for back pain rose by 104 per cent, and it still rises annually. This is coupled with the fact that there is no evidence of an increasing frequency of physical trauma or other organic cause (Potter, 1998). It would thus appear something is going very wrong indeed.

The influence of litigation

Some of the most extensive work on the possible influence of one of these subtle 'secondary gains' was carried out in the mid-1980s. Research was undertaken looking at the influence that adversarial compensation litigation might have on long-term outcome following an acute injury. It would appear that for syndromes such as late whiplash, a cervical sprain syndrome usually occurring following a rear-end collision road traffic accident, the long-term outlook is influenced by the compensation system that is in place within the country rather than by biophysiological factors. Fascinating data can be obtained by reading Mills and Horne's (1986) study comparing the characteristics of whiplash injuries in New Zealand, where a universal system of compensation for injuries exists, with a state in Australia where claimants need to prove injury and suffering in court.

Most of the literature suggests that continuing compensation payments may be a factor in maintaining symptoms and promoting dependency. Some research advocates the need to advise patients to return to work. Although this invariably meets with a very angry response, it is argued that this approach is an important part of overall treatment for patients with chronic pain receiving workers' compensation (Catchlove and Cohen, 1983). A previous study by Catchlove and Cohen in 1982 found that 60 per cent of patients who were told that returning to work was an integral part of their treatment managed to return to the workforce. Only 25 per cent of those with whom these issues were not raised managed to achieve a return to work. When compensation claims are protracted and adversarial, they can only add to the stress associated with chronic pain and injury.

Patients with chronic low back pain with symptoms incongruent with physical findings could well be engaged in less effective coping styles, catastrophising, feeling less in control and displaying extremely compromised physical functioning. A study by Reesor and Craig (1988) looked at 40 patients with such symptoms. They concluded that these patients were often erroneously labelled as malingering simply because no obvious pathological cause for their pain was established. Because patients then felt disbelieved, they might have exaggerated their pain expression in an attempt to convince clinicians that their pain was real. The authors concluded, however, that pending litigation and compensation were not associated with incongruent pain.

Activity

Have you looked after a patient who was receiving, or attempting to claim, compensation following some work-related injury?

What sort of job did he or she have: was it absorbing and interesting, or was it boring and repetitive?

Relief from responsibility, poor job satisfaction and high mental stress

Recent evidence also suggests that psychosocial factors, particularly for conditions such as low back pain, have an influence as great, if not greater, on disability as on ergonomic aspects (Symonds *et al.*, 1996). A job that is perceived as unrewarding and repetitive may significantly impact on an individual's desire to continue with that work. Much more research is needed to unravel the complex associations between negative attitudes and beliefs within the workplace, and extended absence with low back pain. There is, however, some literature that seems to indicate that reports of low back pain can be related, in some instances, to poor job satisfaction and mental stress within the work environment (Bigos *et al.*, 1991).

The influence of the family

Family, friends and carers may unwittingly play a part in perpetuating disability. When we are ill, especially when we are admitted to hospital, we receive cards, flowers and the solicitous visits of friends and family. Other family members take over chores and relieve us of day-to-day household responsibilities.

For most people, this becomes self-limiting as the acute phase of an illness diminishes, but if chronic pain causes a patient's role to become far more passive and dependent, the altered family dynamics may unwittingly contribute to further disability as family members gradually take over the patient's role. If positive strategies to achieve improved mobility and reinforce 'well' behaviour are not fully understood by the family, rehabilitation programmes can be doomed to failure.

case history

Mrs B is a 56-year-old woman with two daughters in their twenties and a son aged 17. Some years ago, she hurt her back lifting a box at work. She has been left with chronic back pain, which she has been told is the result of a 'slipped disc' and general degeneration of her spine. Mrs B also has mild osteoporosis and is now taking hormone replacement therapy. She has become very bitter at the medical profession's seeming inability to do anything to help her pain.

Mrs B has had surgery and multiple caudal epidural injections, and has been admitted to hospital many times for no active treatment other than pain relief, which never really works. She is frequently taken to the A&E department of her local hospital, and the family call out their general practitioner on a regular basis. Nothing ever satisfactorily controls Mrs B's pain and she now spends most of her time either in bed or lying on the sofa. She feels that all her pain is related to damage to her spine and if she does too much she will only make it worse – especially as her 'bones are fragile' as a result of her osteoporosis. Her family are extremely supportive and concerned, undertaking all the domestic chores between them. Mrs B now rarely goes out, but if she does she uses a wheelchair. She is very depressed, cries frequently and no longer sees her friends, and the family are at their wits' end.

Partial solution: Mrs B is finally admitted into a rehabilitation programme that aims to reduce her dependency on analgesia, improve her quality of life and increase her mobility. She is prescribed an antidepressant and commenced on a programme that sets goals on a daily basis in terms of performing tasks and extending her range and scope of mobility, thereby eliminating the need to use aids such as the wheelchair. Mrs B's husband is included in all the patient education components of the programme, and the entire family are urged to substitute 'doing everything' with supporting and encouraging Mrs B to do more for herself.

Such programmes can be very successful in improving patient self-confidence and mobility, thereby reducing disability (see Chapter 9 in Tyrer, 1992) for further text. They never claim to be able to remove pain, but often, as patients become more socially interactive, physically fitter and more confident in their ability to cope with their pain, their quality of life improves. In some cases, it has been reported that the pain has spontaneously resolved.

CONCLUSION

In this chapter, we have discussed the importance of considering other influences, apart from an original pathological cause, that can impact on a person's experience of pain. We have briefly introduced some theories that help to describe how pain sufferers explain or come to terms with the origins of their pain and the extent to which they are prepared to take responsibility for it. A fascinating book that puts forward a different perspective on pain is that by Brand and Yancey (1994); see also Walker *et al.* (1999).

After a break, try the multiple choice questionnaire below in order to self-assess your learning so far.

Suggested further reading

Alleyne, J. and Thomas, V.J. (1994) The management of sickle cell crisis pain as experienced by patients and carers. *Journal of Advanced Nursing*, **19**(4): 725–32.

Beales, J.G. (1982) Factors influencing the expectation of pain among patients in a children's burns unit. *Burns*, **9**(3): 187–92.

Choiniere, M., Melzack, R., Girard, N., Rondeau, J. and Paquin, M.J. (1990) Comparisons between patients' and nurses' assessment of pain and medication efficacy in severe burn injuries. *Pain*, **40**: 143–52.

Cromey, S. (1998) The pain of withdrawing from illicit heroin use. In Carter, B. (ed.) *Perspective on Pain: Mapping the Territory*, London, Arnold, pp. 306–16.

Keefe, K.J., Wilkins, R.H., Cook, W.A., Crisson, J.E. and Muhlbairer, J.H. (1986) Depression, pain and pain behaviour. *Journal of Consulting and Clinical Psychology*, **54**: 665–9.

Litt, M. (1988) Self-efficacy and perceived control: cognitive mediators of pain tolerance. *Journal of Personality and Social Psychology*, **54**: 149–60.

Madjar, I. (1998) *Giving Comfort and Inflicting Pain,* Edmonton, Qual. Institute Press.

Rapp, S.E., Ready, L.B. and Nessly, M.L. (1995) Acute pain management in patients with prior opioid consumption: a case-controlled retrospective review. *Pain,* **61**: 195–201.

Rutledge, D.R. and Donaldson, N.E. (1998) Pain assessment and documentation. Part II – Special populations of adults. *Online Journal of Clinical Innovations,* 1(6): 1–29.

Symons, T.L., Burton, A.K., Tillotson, K.M. and Main, C.J. (1996) Do attitudes and beliefs influence work loss due to low back trouble? *Occupational Medicine,* **46**(1): 25–32.

Thomas, V.N. (ed.) (1997) *Pain: Its Nature and Management,* London, Baillière Tindall. (See Chapter 11).

Waddell, G. (1998) *The Back Pain Revolution.* London, Churchill Livingstone.

Nursing Patients with Challenging Pain

MULTIPLE-CHOICE QUESTIONNAIRE

1. The degree of suffering from burn pain depends upon:

   a. The age of the person as younger children feel less pain due to poorly developed nerve networks ☐

   b. The pain tolerance of an individual ☐

   c. How anxious a person is feeling ☐

   d. It cannot be predicted ☐

2. When assessing pain in people suffering a painful crisis, which is the best approach?

   a. Ask patients to rate their pain on a 1–10 scale ☐

   b. Watch for elevations in blood pressure or pulse rate ☐

   c. Ask patients about their pain and use a rating scale to assess its intensity ☐

   d. Avoid encouraging patients to focus on their pain but observe them for pain behaviours ☐

3. Pain following injury to the spinal cord can usually be divided into two types:

   a. Neurogenic and chronic ☐

   b. Chronic and acute ☐

   c. Nociceptive and neuropathic ☐

   d. Central pain and chronic pain ☐

4. Which of the following people are most at risk of sickle-cell disease?

   a. Caucasians ☐

   b. Asians ☐

   c. Latin Americans ☐

   d. African/Caribbean ☐

MULTIPLE-CHOICE QUESTIONNAIRE (cont'd)

5. When does sickle-cell disease manifest itself and pain become a problem?

   a. In infancy ☐

   b. In adolescence ☐

   c. In young adulthood ☐

   d. In advanced age ☐

6. A regular use of which of the following two drugs will increase tolerance to morphine?

   a. Codeine ☐

   b. An NSAID ☐

   c. Paracetamol ☐

   d. Tramadol ☐

7. Which one of the following opioid drugs could cause withdrawal symptoms in a patient addicted to heroin?

   a. Pethidine ☐

   b. Dihydrocodeine ☐

   c. Buprenorphine ☐

   d. Morphine ☐

8. Which of the following is not normally associated with opioid withdrawal syndrome?

   a. Yawning ☐

   b. Watery eyes ☐

   c. Hypotension ☐

   d. Runny nose ☐

9. You have a heroin addict admitted to your ward with a fractured femur who has also just undergone surgery to remove his spleen. Which of the following goals do you feel is the most important to achieve?

   a. A gradual reduction in opioid dependency ☐

   b. Adequate analgesia involving large doses of opioids ☐

   c. Enrolling the patient onto a drug rehabilitation programme ☐

   d. Avoiding opioids altogether by treating the pain with NSAIDs ☐

10. According to current research patients in pain and attending chronic pain clinics are frequently found to be suffering from which of the following?

   a. Depression ☐

   b. Hypochondriasis ☐

   c. Hysteria ☐

   d. Munchausen syndrome ☐

ANSWERS FOR THE MULTIPLE-CHOICE QUESTIONNAIRE

1. **d. It cannot be predicted**; burns may include a mixture of deep burns (tending to give less pain because of nerve endings being damaged) and superficial burns (often very painful). The age of the person is not significant. Children may need greater reassurance and comfort as they might not be able to respond verbally to pain assessment. All patients who have been burnt will feel pain and the expression of that pain, its meaning for an individual varying depending on a person's tolerance to pain, although many other factors will affect their suffering. The pain experience might be altered by a person's anxiety, but it cannot reliably be said to affect his or her suffering.

2. **c. Ask patients about their pain and use a rating scale to assess its intensity**; this is the best answer as this approach immediately confirms to patients that you are interested in their pain. The rating of pain intensity supplements the data you have collected and can be useful to evaluate the effectiveness of any interventions. With an acute exacerbation of a chronic disease, it is unlikely that a simple pain intensity rating such as the 0–10 scale will tell you very much about the pain. Similarly, with someone who has experienced chronic pain, it is unlikely that physiological parameters will be accurate in reflecting that pain – even with severe pain these may remain 'normal'. Severe pain can sometimes cause 'shock', the blood pressure and pulse rate falling. These are unreliable measures and are best avoided as they can lead to inaccurate conclusions. Encouraging someone to focus on their chronic pain can reduce the effectiveness of distraction strategies. In a painful crisis, however, the pain is very severe and will need regularly assessing to establish analgesia. In this case, it is unlikely that asking patients about their pain will reduce the effectiveness of their coping strategies. Pain behaviours (like physiological behaviours) can be inaccurate predictors of another person's pain experience.

3. **c. Nociceptive and neuropathic**; nociceptive pain is caused by tissue damage, and neuropathic pain by changes in the nervous system itself. The latter might be caused by changes to central (brain or spinal cord) or peripheral structures. Neurogenic pain occurs with tissue damage and is highly likely following a spinal cord injury. Chronic pain is defined as pain that has been present for longer than 3–6 months, which might not always be the case following such an injury. 'Chronic and acute' is incorrect, chronic pain is a broad term for a wide range of pain types. Although it is technically true, it is not sufficiently accurate. Acute pain may or may not be experienced. 'Central pain and chronic pain' is also wrong; central pain is a type of chronic pain, and patients with spinal injury may develop this type of pain – they are both of the same type. The other 'type' of pain is pain caused by tissue damage (nociceptive pain).

4. **d. African/Caribbean**; the condition is most common in this group and is caused by a genetic mutation passed on through certain families.

5. **a. In infancy**; individuals are born with the condition, which is currently incurable.

6. **a and d. Codeine and tramadol** are both pure agonist opioids and provide analgesia predominantly by metabolising to morphine. Neither NSAIDs nor paracetamol would increase tolerance as their actions are both quite different from those of opioids.

7. **c. Buprenorphine**; this is what is termed a partial opioid agonist in that it only partially blocks the opioid receptors. This means that it can block the action of a pure agonist such as morphine or heroin and lead to symptoms of withdrawal. It is difficult to reverse with naloxone for this same reason. All the other drugs on the list are pure agonists.

8. **c. Hypotension** is not normally associated with withdrawal syndrome, although hypertension and an increase in pulse rate are. Yawning, watery eyes and a runny nose are very common symptoms of withdrawal and will often be a valuable clue should a patient be denying withdrawal or staff be unfamiliar with the symptoms.

9. **b. Adequate analgesia involving large doses of opioids** is the most appropriate answer. Although a gradual reduction in opioid dependency and enrolling a patient on a drug rehabilitation programme are very commendable goals to aim for, it is highly unlikely these will be successful once a patient is in hospital and experiencing pain and stress away from his or her usual support strategies; it is probably inappropriate to articulate these goals during the acute phase of the patient's recovery. Treating the pain with NSAIDs alone would almost certainly lead to the patient experiencing painful and distressing withdrawal symptoms.

10. **a. Depression**; there is a higher incidence of depression in chronic pain patients than in patients without pain. In one study, approximately 33 per cent of patients were found to be clinically depressed (Turner and Romano, 1984). Very little research has been undertaken to look at the incidences of hypochondriasis and hysteria (terms currently losing favour) or Munchausen syndrome.

References

Chapter 1

Brescia, F.J., Portenoy, R.K., Ryan, M., Krasnoff, L. and Gray, G. (1992) Pain, opioid use, and survival in hospitalised patients with advanced cancer. *Journal of Oncology*, **10**: 149–55.

Bruster, S., Jarman, B., Bosanquet, N., Weston, D., Erens, R. and Delbanco, T.L. (1994) National survey of hospital patients. *British Medical Journal*, **309**: 1542–6.

Carr, D.B. and Goudas, L.C. (1999) Acute pain. *Lancet*, **353**: 2051–8.

Collin, E., Poulain, P., Gauvain-Piquard, A. *et al.* (1993) Is disease progression the major factor in morphine 'tolerance' in cancer pain treatment? *Pain*, **55**: 319–26.

Dubner, R., and Ruda, M.A. (1992) Activity-dependent neuronal plasticity following tissue injury and inflammation. *Trends in Neurosciences*, **15**: 96–103.

Egbert, A.M., Battit, G.E., Welch, C.E. and Bartlett, M.K. (1964) Reduction of postoperative pain by encouragement and instruction of patients. *New England Journal of Medicine*, **270**: 825–7.

Elliott, T.E. and Elliott, B.A. (1992) Physicians' attitudes and beliefs about use of morphine for cancer pain. *Journal of Pain and Symptom Management*, **7**: 141–8.

Ferrell, B.R., McCaffery, M. and Rhiner, M. (1992) Pain and addiction: an urgent need for change in nursing education. *Journal of Pain and Symptom Management*, **7**(2): 117–24.

Foley, K.M. (1993) Pain assessment and cancer pain syndromes. In Doyle, D., Hanks G.W.C. and MacDonald N. (eds) *Oxford Textbook of Palliative Medicine*, Oxford, Oxford Medical Publications, Chapter 4.

Friedman, D.P. (1990) Perspectives on the medical use of drug abuse. *Journal of Pain and Symptom Management*, **5**: S2–S5.

Gracely, R.H., Lynch, S.A. and Bennett, G.J. (1992) Painful neuropathy: altered central processing maintained dynamically by peripheral input. *Pain*, **51**: 175–94.

Hayward, J. (1975) *Information: A Prescription Against Pain*, London, RCN.

International Association for the Study of Pain (1986) Classification of chronic pain. Descriptions of chronic pain syndromes and definitions of pain terms. *Pain* (Supplement 3): S1–S226.

Leibeskind, J.C. and Melzack, R. (1987) The international pain foundation: meeting a need for education in pain management. *Pain*, **30**: 1–2.

Loeb, J. (1999) Pain management in long-term care. *American Journal of Nursing*, **99**(2): 48–52.

McCaffery, M. (1968) *Nursing practice theories related to cognition, bodily pain and non-environment interactions*, Los Angeles, University of California.

McCaffery, M. (1979) *Nursing Management of the Patient with Pain*, New York, J.B. Lippincott, pp. 137–83.

McCaffery, M. and Beebe, A. (1994) *Pain: A Clinical Manual of Nursing Practice*, London, C.V. Mosby.

McCaffery, M., Ferrell, B., O'Neil-Page, E. and Lester, M. (1990) Nurses' knowledge of opioid analgesic drugs and psychological dependence. *Cancer Nursing*, **13**: 21–7.

McQuay, H.J. (1999) Opioids in pain management. *Lancet*, **353**: 2229–32.

McQuay, H.J. and Dickenson, A.H. (1990) Implication of nervous system plasticity for pain management. *Anaesthesia*, **45**: 101–2.

Melzack, R. and Wall, P. (1965) Pain mechanisms: a new theory. *Science*, **150**: 971–9.

Melzack, R. and Wall, P. (1982) *The Challenge of Pain*, New York, Basic Books.

Melzack, R. and Wall, P. (1999) *Textbook of Pain*, 4th edn, Edinburgh, Churchill Livingstone.

Porter, J. and Jick, H. (1980) Addiction rare in patients treated with narcotics. *New England Journal of Medicine*, **301**: 419–26.

Sluka, K.A. and Rees, H. (1997) The neuronal response to pain. *Physiotherapy Theory and Practice*, **13**(1): 3–22.

Twycross, R. and Lack, S. (1989) *Oral Morphine in Advanced Cancer*, 2nd edn, Beaconsfield, Beaconsfield Publishers.

Waddell, G. (1997) Low back pain: a twentieth century health care enigma. In Jensen, T.S., Turner, A. and Weisenfeld-Hallin, Z. (eds) *Progress in Pain Research and Management*, vol. 8. Seattle, International Association for the Study of Pain, pp. 101–12.

Wall, P. (1999) *The Science of Suffering*, London, Weidenfeld & Nicolson.

Chapter 2

Allcock, N. (1996) Factors affecting the assessment of postoperative pain: a literature review. *Journal of Advanced Nursing*, **24**: 1144–51.

Baillie, L. (1993) A review of pain assessment tools. *Nursing Standard*, **7**(23): 25–9.

Briggs, M. (1995) Principles of acute pain assessment. *Nursing Standard*, **9**(19): 23–7.

Bush, F.M., Harkins, S.W., Harrington, W.G. and Price, D.D. (1993) Analysis of gender effects on pain perception and symptom presentation in temporomandibular pain. *Pain*, **53**: 73–80.

Camp, D.L. and O'Sullivan, P. (1987) Comparison of surgical and oncology patients' descriptions of pain and nurses' documentation of pain assessments. *Journal of Advanced Nursing*, **12**: 593–8.

Carr, E.C.J. (1997a) Evaluating the use of a pain assessment tool and care plan – a pilot study. *Journal of Advanced Nursing*, **26**(6): 1073–9.

Carr, E.C.J. (1997b) Overcoming barriers to effective pain control. *Professional Nurse*, **12**(6): 412–16.

Feine, J.S. Bushell, M.M., Miron, D. and Duncan G.H. (1991) Sex differences in the perception of noxious heat stimuli. *Pain*, **44**: 255–62.

Francke A.L. and Theeuwen, I. (1994) Inhibition in expressing pain: a qualitative study among Dutch surgical breast cancer patients. *Cancer Nursing*, **17**(3): 193–9.

Harrison, A. (1991) Assessing patients' pain: identifying reasons for error. *Journal of Advanced Nursing*, **16**: 1018–25.

Hayes, R. (1995) Pain assessment in the elderly. *British Journal of Nursing*, **4**(20): 1199–204.

Latham, J. (1989) *Pain Control*, London, Austin Cornish.

McCaffery, M. (1991) Pain control vignettes: how would you respond to these patients in pain? *Nursing*, **21**(6): 34–7.

Melzack, R. (1987) The short-form McGill Pain Questionnaire. *Pain*, **30**: 191–7.

Melzack, R. and Katz, J. (1994) Pain measurement in persons in pain. In Wall, P.D. and Melzack, R. (eds) *Textbook of Pain*, 3rd edn, Edinburgh, Churchill Livingstone, pp. 337–56.

Melzack, R. and Torgerson, W. (1971) On the language of pain. *Anaesthesiology*, **34**(1): 50–9.

Nagy, S. (1998) A comparison of the effects of patients' pain on nurses working in burns and neonatal intensive care units. *Journal of Advanced Nursing*, **27**(2): 335–40.

Raiman, J. (1986) Pain relief – a two way process. *Nursing Times*, **82**(15): 24–7.

Seers, K. (1987) Perceptions of pain. *Nursing Times*, **83**: 37–9.

Shade, P. (1992) PCA: can client education improve outcomes? *Journal of Advanced Nursing*, **17**: 408–13.

Zalon, M.L. (1993) Nurses' assessment of postoperative patients' pain. *Pain*, **54**: 329–34.

Chapter 3

Agency for Health Care Policy and Research (1992) *Acute Pain Management*. Publication No. 92–0032, Rockville, MD, Department of Health and Human Services.

Audit Commission (1997) *Anaesthesia Under Examination*, London, Audit Commission.

Ballantyne, J.C., Carr, D.B., Chalmers, T.C., Dear, K.G.B. and Angellilo, I.F. (1993) Postoperative patient controlled analgesia: meta analyses of initial randomised controlled trials. *Journal of Clinical Anaesthesiology*, **5**: 182–93.

Blair, J.S. (1967) Phenazocine hydrobromide BPC in the management of incurable malignant disease. *British Journal of Clinical Practice*, **21**(3): 124–6.

Brockopp, D.Y., Brockopp, G., Warden, S., Wilson, J., Carpenter, J.S. and Vandeveer, B. (1998) Barriers to change: a pain management project. *International Journal of Nursing Studies*, **35**: 226–32.

Bruster, S., Jarman, B., Bosanquet, N., Weston, D., Erens, R. and Delbanco, T.L. (1994) National survey of hospital patients. *British Medical Journal*, **309**: 1542–6.

Carr, D. and Goudas, L. (1999) Acute pain. *Lancet*, **353**: 2051–8.

Carr, E.C.J. and Thomas, V.J. (1997) Anticipating and experiencing postoperative pain: the patients' perspective. *Journal of Clinical Nursing*, **6**(3): 191–201.

Dahl, J.B., Rosenberg, J., Dirkes, W.E., Mogensen, T. and Kehlet, H. (1990) Prevention of postoperative pain by balanced analgesia. *British Journal of Anaesthesia*, **64**: 518–20.

Donovan, M. (1990) Acute pain relief. *Nursing Clinics of North America*, **25**(4): 851–61.

Economou G., Monson, R. and Ward-McQuaid, J.N. (1971) Oral pentazocine and phenazocine: a comparison in postoperative pain. *British Journal of Anaesthesia*, **43**(5): 486–94.

Evans, J.M.M., McMahon, A., McGilchrist, M. et al. (1995) Topical non-steroidal anti-inflammatory drugs and admission to hospital for upper gastrointestinal bleeding and perforation: a record lineage case-control study. British Medical Journal, 311: 22–6.

Friedman, D.P. (1990) Perspectives on the medical use of drug abuse. Journal of Pain and Symptom Management, 5: S2–S5.

Good, M. (1996) Effects of relaxation and music on postoperative pain: a review. Journal of Advanced Nursing, 24: 905–14.

Griepp, M. (1992) Undermedication for pain: an ethical model. Advances in Nursing Science, 15(1): 44–53.

Hargreaves, A. and Lander, J. (1989) Use of transcutaneous electrical nerve stimulation for postoperative pain. Nursing Research, 38(3): 159–61.

International Association for the Study of Pain (1986) Classification of chronic pain. Descriptions of chronic pain syndromes and definitions of pain terms. Pain, (Supplement 3): S216.

Jaques, A. (1994) Epidural analgesia. British Journal of Nursing, 3(14): 734–8.

Jayson, M.I.V. (1997) Why does acute back pain become chronic (editorial). British Medical Journal, 314: 1639.

Jones, M. (1998) 'Acute pain teams: the future (guest editorial). Acute Pain, 1(3): 5–6.

Kehlet, H. (1997) Multimodal approach to control postoperative pathophysiology and rehabilitation. British Journal of Anaesthesia, 78: 606–17.

Koh, P. and Thomas, V.J. (1994) Patient-controlled analgesia (PCA): does time saved by PCA improve patient satisfaction with nursing care? Journal of Advanced Nursing, 20: 61–70.

Linton, S.J. (1994) Chronic back pain: integrating psychological and physical therapy: an overview. Behavioural Medicine, 20: 101–4.

McCaffery, M. and Beebe, A. (1994) Pain: A Clinical Manual for Nursing Practice, London, C.V. Mosby.

McQuay, H. (1999) Opioids in pain management. Lancet, 353: 2229–32.

McQuay H., and Moore, A. (1998) An Evidence-based Resource for Pain Relief, Oxford, Oxford University Press.

McQuay, H., Moore, A. and Justins, D. (1997) Treating acute pain in hospital. British Medical Journal, 314: 1531–5.

Madjar, I. (1998) Giving Comfort and Inflicting Pain, Edmonton, Qual Institute Press.

Mather, C.M.P. and Ready, L.B. (1994) Management of acute pain. British Journal of Hospital Medicine, 51(3): 85–8.

Nagle, C.J. and McQuay, H. (1990) Opioid receptors; their role in effect and side-effect. Current Anaesthesia and Critical Care, 1: 247–52.

Needleman, P. and Isakson, P.C. (1998) Selective inhibition of cyclo-oxygenase 2. Science and Medicine, Jan./Feb.: 26–35.

Notcutt, W. (1997) Better to define and enhance the role of ward surgical nurses (letter). British Medical Journal, 314: 1347.

Ready, L.B., Oden, R., Chadwick, H.S. et al. (1988) Development of an anaesthesiology-based postoperative pain management service. Anaesthesiology, 68: 100–6.

Royal College of Anaesthetists (1998) *Clinical Guidelines: Guidelines for the Use of Non-steroidal Anti-inflammatory Drugs in the Perioperative Period*, Oxford, Royal College of Anaesthetists.

Royal College of Surgeons and College of Anaesthetists (1990) *Report of the Working Party on Pain after Surgery*, London, HMSO.

Smith, G. (1998) Audit and bridging the analgesic gap (editorial). *Anaesthesia*, **53**: 521–2.

Spencer, L., Carpenter, R.L. and Neal, J.M. (1995) Epidural anaesthesia and analgesia – their role in postoperative outcome. *Anaesthesiology*, **82**(6): v.

Stevenson, C. (1995) Non-pharmacological aspects of acute pain management. *Complementary Therapies in Nursing and Midwifery*, **1**: 77–84.

Tasmuth, T., Estlanderb, A. and Kalso, E. (1996) Effect of present and mood on the memory of past postoperative pain in women treated surgically for breast cancer. *Journal of Advanced Nursing*, **68**: 343–5.

Taylor, N.M., Hall, G.M. and Salmon, P. (1996) Patients' experiences of patient-controlled analgesia. *Anaesthesia*, **51**: 525–8.

Thomas, V.J. (1993) Patient and staff perceptions of PCA. *Nursing Standard*, **7**(28): 37–9.

Thomas, V.J. and Rose, F.D. (1993) Patient-controlled analgesia: a new method for old. *Journal of Advanced Nursing*, **18**: 1719–26.

Waddell, G. (1992) Biopsychosocial analysis of low back pain. *Baillière's Clinical Rheumatology*. **6**: 523–51.

Welchew, E. (1995) *Patient Controlled Analgesia*, London, BMJ Publishing Group.

Windsor, A.L.M., Glynn, C.J. and Mason, D.G. (1996) National provision of pain services. *Anaesthesia*, **51**: 228–31.

World Health Organization (1996) *Cancer Pain Relief*, 2nd edn, Geneva, World Health Organization.

Chapter 4

Albrecht, M.N., Cook, J.E., Riley, M.J. and Andreoni, V. (1992) Factors influencing staff nurses' decisions for non-documentation of patient response to analgesia administration. *Journal of Clinical Nursing*, **1**: 243–51.

Backonja, M., Beydoun, A., Edwards, K. *et al.* (1998) Gabapentin for the symptomatic treatment of painful neuropathy in patients with diabetes mellitus: a randomised controlled trial. *Journal of the American Medical Association*, **280**: 1831–6.

Barsoum, G., Perry, E.P., Fraser I.A. *et al.* (1990) Postoperative nausea is relieved by acupressure. *Journal of the Royal Society of Medicine*, **83**: 86–9.

Bates, M.S., Edwards, W.T. and Anderson, K.O. (1993) Ethnocultural influences on variation in chronic pain perception. *Pain*, **52**: 101–12.

Bill, K., and Dundee, J. (1988) Acupressure for postoperative nausea and vomiting. *British Journal of Clinical Pharmacology*, **26**: 225.

Carroll D. (1997) A non-pharmacological approach to chronic pain. *Professional Nurse Study* (Supplement) **13**(1): S12–S14.

Christensen, J. (1993) *Nursing Partnership: A Model for Nursing Practice*, Edinburgh, Churchill Livingstone.

Crabbe, G. (1989) Crossing the pain threshold. *Nursing Times*, **85**(47): 16–17.

Deardorff, W.W., Robin, H.S. and Scott, D.W. (1991) Comprehensive multidisciplinary treatment of chronic pain: a follow-up study of treated and non-treated groups. *Pain*, **145**: 35–43.

Good, M. (1996) Effects of relaxation and music on postoperative pain: a review. *Journal of Advanced Nursing*, **24**: 905–14.

Glynn, C.J., McQuay, H.J., Jahad, A.J. and Carroll, D. (1991) Response to controversy corner: opioids in patients with non-malignant pain. Questions in search of answers. *Clinical Journal of Pain*, **7**(4): 346.

Hill, A., Niven, C.A. and Knussen, C. (1995) The role of coping adjustment to phantom limb pain. *Pain*, **62**: 79–86.

International Association for the Study of Pain (1986) Classification of chronic pain. Descriptions of chronic pain syndromes and definitions of pain terms. *Pain* (Supplement 3): S1–S226.

Jacox, A., Carr, D.B., Payne, R. *et al.* (1994) *Management of Cancer Pain*. Clinical Practice Guideline No. 9, AHCPR Pub. No. 94–0592, M D Agency for Health Care Policy and Research, Washington, US Department of Health and Human Services, Public Health Service.

King, V.M.F. and Jacob, P.A. (1993) Special procedures. In Carroll, D. and Bowsher, D. (eds) *Pain: Management and Nursing Care*, Oxford, Butterworth-Heinemann, pp. 206–47.

McCaffery, M. and Beebe, A. (1989) *Pain: Clinical Manual for Nursing Practice*, St Louis, C.V. Mosby.

McQuay, H.J., Moore, R.A., Eccleston, C., Morley, S. and Williams, A.C. (1997) Systematic review of outpatient services for chronic pain control. *Health Technology Assessment*, **1**(6): 1–236.

McQuay, H.J., Tramer, M., Nye, B.A., Carroll, D., Wiffen, P.J. and Moore, R.A. (1996) A systematic review of antidepressants in neuropathic pain. *Pain*, **68**: 217–27.

Mann, E.M. (1999) Using acupuncture and acupressure to treat postoperative emesis. *Professional Nurse*, **14**(10): 691–4.

Ochs, G., Struppler, A., Meyerson, B.A. *et al.* (1989) Intrathecal baclofen for long-term treatment of spasticity: multi-centre study. *Journal of Neurology, Neurosurgery and Psychiatry*, **52**: 933–9.

O'Hara, P. (1996) The role of the professionals. In O'Hara, P. *Pain Management for Health Professionals*, London, Chapman & Hall, pp. 122–41.

Penn, R.D., Savoy, S.M., Corcos, D.M. *et al.* (1989) Intrathecal baclofen for severe spinal spasticity. *New England Journal of Medicine*, **23**: 1517–21.

Phillips, K. and Leicester, G. (1993) A point of pressure. *Nursing Times*, **89**(45): 44–5.

Potter, R.G. (1990) The frequency of presentation of pain in general practice: an analysis of 1000 consecutive consultations. *Journal of the Pain Society*, **8**: 112–16.

Potter, R.G. (1998) The prevention of chronic pain. In Carter, B. (ed.) *Perspectives on Pain: Mapping the Territory*, London, Arnold, pp. 186–94.

Quan, D.B. and Wandres, D.L. (1993) Clonodine in pain management. *Annals of Pharmacotherapy*, **27**: 313–15.

Richardson, A. (1997) Cancer pain and its management. In V.N. Thomas (ed.) *Pain: Its Nature and Management*, London, Baillière Tindall. pp. 194–219.

Rowbotham, M., Harden, M., Stacey, B. and Bernstein, P. (1998) Gabapentin for the treatment of postherpetic neuralgias: a randomized controlled trial. *Journal of the American Medicine Association*, **280**: 1837–42.

Seers, K. (1997) Chronic non-malignant pain: a community-based approach to management. In Thomas, V.J. (ed.) *Pain: Its Nature and Management*, London, Baillière Tindall, pp. 220–37.

Seers, K. and Friedli, K. (1996) The patients' experiences of their chronic non-malignant pain. *Journal of Advanced Nursing*, **24**: 1160–8.

Stevenson, C. (1995) Non-pharmacological aspects of acute pain management. *Complementary Therapies in Nursing and Midwifery*, **1**: 77–84.

Waddell, G. (1992) Biopsychosocial analysis of low back pain. *Baillière's Clinical Rheumatology*, **6**: 523–51.

Walker, J., Davis, B.D. and Marcer, D. (1989) The nursing management of pain in the community: a theoretical framework. *Journal of Advanced Nursing*, **14**: 240, 247.

Walsh, D. (1997) *TENS – Clinical Applications and Related Theory*, Edinburgh, Churchill Livingstone.

Williams, A. (1997) Psychological techniques in the management of pain. In Thomas V.N. (ed.) *Pain: Its Nature and Management*, London, Baillière Tindall, pp. 108–24.

Chapter 5

Brockopp, D.Y., Brockopp, G., Warden, S., Wilson, J., Carpenter, J.S. and Vandeveer, B. (1998) Barrier to change: a pain management project. *International Journal of Nursing Studies*, **35**: 226–32.

Carr, E.C.J. and Mann, E.M. (1998) *Partnering Patients to Manage Pain after Surgery*, Bournemouth, Institute of Health and Community Studies, Bournemouth University.

Carr, E.C.J. and Thomas, V.J. (1997) Anticipating and experiencing postoperative pain: the patients' perspective. *Journal of Clinical Nursing*, **6**(3): 191–210.

Clarke, E.B., French, B., Bilodeau, M.L., Capasso, V.C., Edwards, A. and Empoliti, J. (1996) Pain management knowledge, attitudes and clinical practice: the impact of nurses' characteristics and education. *Journal of Pain and Symptom Management*, **11**(1): 18–31.

Closs, S.J. (1996) Pain and elderly patients: a survey of nurses' knowledge and experiences. *Journal of Advanced Nursing*, **23**: 237–42.

Crown, J. (1999) Review of prescribing, supply and administration of medicines. Final report, London, DoH.

Department of Health (1991) *The Patient's Charter*, London, HMSO.

Department of Health (1998) *The New National Health Service*, London, HMSO.

Fagerhaugh, S.Y. and Strauss, A. (1977) *Politics of Pain Management: Staff–Patient Interaction*, London, Addison-Wesley.

Franke, A.L., Garssen, B. and Abu-Saad, H.H. (1996) Continuing pain education in nursing: a literature review. *International Journal of Nursing Studies*, **33**(5): 567–78.

Funnell, P. (1995) Exploring the value of interprofessional shared learning. In Soothill, K. Mackay, L. and Webb, C. (eds) *Interprofessional Relations in Health Care*, London, Edward Arnold, pp. 163–71.

Gabrielczyk, M.R. (1995) Low expectations of pain relief encourage persistence of poor standards. *British Medical Journal*, **311**: 1024.

General Medical Council (1997) *The New Doctor*, London, GMC.

Graffam, S. (1990) Pain Content in the Curriculum: A Survey. *Nurse Educator*, **15**(1): 20–3.

Greipp, M.E. (1992) Undermedication for pain: an ethical model. *Advances in Nursing Science*, **15**(1): 44–53.

Jacox, A., Ferrell, B. and Heidrich, G. (1992) Managing acute pain: a guideline for the nation. *American Journal of Nursing*, **92**(5): 49–55.

Lander, J. (1990) Clinical judgements in pain management. *Pain*, **42**: 15–22.

McCaffery, M., Ferrel, B. and Page, E. (1990) Nurses' knowledge of opioid analgesic drugs and psychological dependence. *Cancer Nursing*, **13**(1): 21–7.

McGettrick, S. and Rogers, J. (1996) Cost of administering controlled drugs in a hospice ward. *Health Bulletin*, **54**(6): 441–3.

McQuay, H., Moore, A. and Justins, D. (1997) Clinical review: treating pain in hospital. *British Medical Journal*, **314**: 1531–5.

Marcer, D. and Deighton, S. (1988) Intractable pain: a neglected area of medical education in the U.K. *Journal of the Royal Society of Medicine*, **81**: 698–700.

Marks, R. and Sachar, E. (1973) The undertreatment of medical inpatients with narcotic analgesia. *Annals of Internal Medicine*, **78**: 173–81.

Michaud, G. (1970) *Problems of Teaching Research in University*, Paris, OECD.

Moores, Y. (1999) Clinical governance and nursing. *Professional Nurse*, **15**(2): 74–5.

Morgan, J. (1985) American opioidphobia: customary under-utilisation of opioid analgesics. *Advances in Alcohol Substance Abuse*, **5**: 163–73.

NHS Executive (1999) *Clinical Governance: Quality in the New NHS*. London, Department of Health.

Pearson, A. (ed.) (1988) *Primary Nursing*, London, Croom Helm.

Poyhia, R. and Kalso, E. (1991) Pain related undergraduate teaching in medical faculties in Finland. *Pain*, **79**: 121–5.

Reisner, S.J. (1993) The era of the patient: using the experience of illness in shaping the missions of health care. *Journal of the American Medical Association*, **269**(8): 1012–17.

Royal College of Surgeons and College of Anaesthetists (1990) *Report of the Working Party on Pain after Surgery*, London, HMSO.

Scott, N.B. and Hodson, M. (1997) Public perceptions of postoperative pain and its relief. *Anaesthesia*, **52**: 438–42.

UKCC (1992) *Code of Professional Conduct*, London, UKCC.

Vortherms, R., Ryan, P. and Ward, S. (1992) Knowledge of, attitudes towards, and barriers to pharmacological management of cancer pain in a statewide random sample of nurses. *Research in Nursing and Health*, **15**: 459–66.

Wallace, K.G., Graham, K.M., Ventura, M.R. and Burke, R. (1997) Lesson learned in implementing a staff education program in pain management in the acute care setting. *Journal of Nursing Staff Development*, **13**(1): 24–31.

White, R. (1985) Policy implications and constraints in the role of the nurse in the management of pain. In Copp, L.A. (ed.) *Perspectives on Pain: Recent Advances in Nursing*, Edinburgh, Churchill Livingstone, pp. 75–91.

Winefield, H.R., Katsikitis, M., Hart, L. and Rounsefell, B.F. (1990) Postoperative pain experiences and relevant patient and staff attitudes. *Journal of Psychosomatic Research*, **34**(5): 543–52.

Chapter 6

Ahles, T.A., Cohen, R.E., Little, D., Balducci, L., Dubbert, P.M. and Keane, R.M. (1984) Toward a behavioural assessment of anticipatory symptoms associated with cancer chemotherapy. *Journal of Behaviour Therapy and Experimental Psychiatry*, **15**(2): 141–5.

Anderson, K.O., Bradley, L.A., Turner, R.A. *et al.* (1992) Observation of pain behaviour in rheumatoid arthritis patients during physical examination. Relationship to disease activity and psychological variables. *Arthritis Care and Research*, **5**(1): 49–56.

Baker, A., Bowring, L., Brignell, A. and Kafford, D. (1996) Chronic pain management in cognitively impaired patients: a preliminary research project. *Perspectives*, **2**(20): 4–8.

Beck, M. (1988) *The Theory and Practice of Therapeutic Massage*, New York, Milady.

Billmire, D.A., Neale, N.W. and Gregory, R.O. (1985) Use of i.v. fentanyl in the outpatient treatment of paediatric facial trauma. *Journal of Trauma*, **25**(11): 1079–80.

Bowler, I.M.W. (1993) Stereotypes of women of Asian descent in midwifery: some evidence. *Midwifery*, **9**(1): 7–16.

Choiniere, M., Melzack, R. and Paquin, M.J. (1990) Comparisons between patients' nurses' assessment of pain and medication efficacy in severe burn injuries. *Pain*, **40**: 143–52.

Closs, A.J. (1994) Pain in elderly patients: a neglected phenomenon? *Journal of Advanced Nursing*, **19**: 1072–81.

Collins (1987) *Dictionary and Thesaurus in One Volume*, London, HarperCollins.

Corran, T.M. and Melita, B. (1998) Pain in later life. In Carter, B. (ed.) *Perspectives on Pain: Mapping The Territory*, London, Arnold, pp. 243–63.

Crombie, I., Croft, P., Linton, S., Leresche, L. and Von Korff, M. (1999) *Epidemiology of Pain*, Seattle, IASP Press.

Davitz, L.L. and Davitz, J.R. (1985) Culture and nurses' inferences of suffering. In Copp, L.A. (ed.) *Recent Advances in Nursing (Perspectives on Pain)*, Edinburgh, Churchill Livingstone, pp. 17–28.

Davitz, L.L. and Pendleton, S.H. (1969) Nurses' inferences of suffering. *Nursing Research*, **18**: 100–7.

Department of Health (1991) *The Patient's Charter*, London, HMSO.

Dieppe, P. (1987) Osteoarthritis and related disorders. In Wetherall, D.J., Ledingham, J.G.G. and Warrell, D.A. (eds) *Oxford Textbook of Medicine*, 2nd edn, Oxford, Oxford Medical Publications, pp. 76–84.

Farrell, M.J., Gibson, S.J. and Helme, R.D. (1996) Chronic non-malignant pain in older people. In Ferrell, B.R. and Ferrell, B.A. (eds) *Pain in the Elderly*, Seattle, IASP Press, pp. 81–9.

Fitzgerald, M. and Koltzenburg, M. (1986) The function development of descending inhibitory pathways in the dorsolateral funiculus of the newborn rat spinal cord. *Developmental Brain Research*, **24**: 261–70.

Flaskerud, J.H. (ed.) (1999) Emerging nursing care of vulnerable populations. *Nursing Clinics of North America*, **34**(2): xv–xvi.

Forrest, D. (1989) The experience of caring. *Journal of Advanced Nursing*, **14**: 815–23.

Franck, L.S. (1986) A new method to quantitatively describe pain behaviour in infants. *Nursing Research*, **35**(1): 28–31.

Frank, A.J.M., Moll, J.M.H. and Hart, J.F. (1992) A comparison of three ways of measuring pain. *Rheumatology and Rehabilitation*, **21**: 211–17.

Gibson, S.J. and Helme, R.D. (1995) Age difference in pain perception and report: a review of physiological, psychological, laboratory and clinical studies. In Budd, K. and Hamann, W. (eds) *Pain Reviews,* vol. 2, London, Edward Arnold, pp. 111–37.

Hawthorn, J. and Redmond, K. (1998) *Pain: Causes and Management*, London, Blackwell Science.

Helme, R.D., Katz, B., Neufeld, M., Lachal, S., Herbert, J. and Conran, T. (1989) The establishment of a geriatric pain clinic: a preliminary report of the first 100 patients. *Australian Journal of Ageing*, **8**: 27–30.

Horgan, M., Choonara, I., Al-Waidh, M., Sambrooks, J. and Ashby, D. (1996) Measuring pain in neonates: an objective score. *Paediatric Nursing*, **8**(10): 24–7.

Jerrett, M.D. (1985) Children and their pain experience. *Children's Health Care*, **14**: 83–9.

Kanarek, R.B., White, E.S., Biegen, M.T. and Kaufman, R. (1991) Cited in Lewindon, P.J., Harkness, L. and Lewindon, N. (1998) Randomised controlled trial of sucrose by mouth for the relief of infant crying after immunisation. *Archives of Disease in Childhood*, **78**: 453–6.

Keefe, F.J. and Block, A.R. (1982) Development of an observation method for assessing pain behaviour in chronic low back pain patients. *Behaviour Therapy*, **13**: 363–75.

Krechel, S.W. and Bilner, J. (1995) CRIES: a new neonatal postoperative pain measurement score. Initial testing of validity and reliability. *Paediatric Anaesthesia*, **5**: 53–61.

Lewindon, P.J., Harkness, L. and Lewindon, N. (1998) Randomised controlled trial of sucrose by mouth for the relief of infant crying after immunisation. *Archives of Disease in Childhood*, **78**: 453–6.

Liebeskind, J.C. and Melzack, R. (1987) The international pain foundation: meeting a need for education in pain management. *Pain*, **30**: 1.

McGrath, P.J., Johnson, G., Goodman, J.T., Schillinger, J., Dunn, J. and Chapman, J. (1985) CHEOPS: a behavioural scale for rating postoperative pain in children. In Fields, H.L., Dubner, R. and Cervero, F. (eds) *Advances in Pain Research and Therapy*, New York, Raven Press, pp. 395–402.

McGrath, P.A. (1989) Evaluating a child's pain. *Journal of Pain and Symptom Management*, **4**(4): 198–214.

Marzinski, L. (1991) The tragedy of dementia: clinically assessing pain in the confused, non-violent elderly. *Journal of Gerontological Nursing*, **6**(6): 25–8.

Meinhart, N.T. and McCaffery, M. (1983) *Pain: A Nursing Approach to Assessment and Analysis*, Norwalk, CO, Appleton Century Crofts.

Melzack, R. and Wall, P.D. (1996) *The Challenge of Pain*, Harmondsworth, Penguin.

Parmelee, P.A. (1996) Pain in cognitively impaired older persons. In Ferrell, B.A. (ed.) *Clinics in Geriatric Medicine: Pain Management*, Philadelphia, W.B. Saunders, pp. 473–87.

Roy, R. and Thomas, M. (1986) A survey of chronic pain in elderly populations. *Canadian Family Physician*, **32**: 513–16.

Royal College of Nursing (1999) *UK Guidelines and Implementation Guide*, London, RCN Publishing.

Sengstaken, E.A. and King, S.A. (1993) The problems of pain and its detection among geriatric nursing home residents. *Journal of the American Geriatric Society*, **41**: 541–4.

Simons, W. and Malabar, R. (1995) Assessing pain in elderly patients who cannot respond verbally. *Journal of Advanced Nursing*, **22**: 663–9.

Tarbel, S.E., Cohen, I.T. and Marsh, J.L. (1992) The toddler–pre-schooler postoperative pain scale: an observational scale for measuring postoperative pain in children aged 1–5. Preliminary report. *Pain*, **50**: 273–80.

Teske, K., Daut, R.L. and Cleeland, C.S. (1983) Relationships between nurses' observations and patients' self-reports of pain. *Pain*, **16**(3): 289–96.

Valman, H.B. and Pearson, J.F. (1980) What the foetus feels. *British Medical Journal*, **280**: 233–4.

Wall, P.D. and Jones, M. (1991) *Defeating Pain: The War against a Silent Epidemic*, New York, Plenum Press.

Zborowski, M. (1952) Cultural components and responses to pain. Cited in Hawthorn, J. and Redmond, K. (1998) *Pain: Causes and Management*, London, Blackwell Science, p. 83.

Zhang, T., Reid, D.K., Acuff, C.G., Jin, D.B. and Rochold, R.W. (1994) Cited in Lewindon, P.J., Harkness, L. and Lewindon, N. (1998) Randomised controlled trial of sucrose by mouth for the relief of infant crying after immunisation. *Archives of Disease in Childhood*, **78**: 453–6.

Chapter 7

Alleyne, J. and Thomas, V.J. (1994) The management of sickle cell crisis pain as experienced by patients and their carers. *Journal of Advanced Nursing*, **19**(4): 725–32.

American Pain Society (1989) Cited in McCaffery, M. and Vourakis, C. (1992) Assessment and relief of pain in chemically dependent patients. *Orthopaedic Nursing*, **11**(2): 13–27.

American Psychiatric Association (1987) Cited in McCaffery, M., and Vourakis, C. (1992) Assessment and relief of pain in chemical dependent patients. *Orthopaedic Nursing*, **11**(2): 13–27.

Atkinson, A. (1998) Nursing burn wounds on general wards. *Nursing Standard*, **12**(41): 58–67.

Bigos, S.J., Battie, M.C., Spengler, D.M. *et al.* (1991) A prospective study of work perceptions and psychosocial factors affecting the report of back injury. *Spine*, **16**: 1–6.

Bowsher, D. (1999) Central pain following spinal and supraspinal injury. *Spinal Cord*, **37**: 235–8.

Brand, P. and Yancey, P. (1994) *Pain: The Gift Nobody Wants*. London, Marshall Pickering.

Catchlove, R. and Cohen, K. (1982) Effects of a directive return to work approach in the treatment of workmen's compensation patients with chronic pain. *Pain*, **14**: 181–91.

Catchlove, R. and Cohen, K. (1983) Directive approach with workmen's compensation patients. *Advances in Pain Research and Therapy*, **5**: 913–18.

Cromey, S. (1998) The pain of withdrawing from illicit heroin use. In Carter, B. (ed.) *Perspectives on Pain: Mapping the Territory*, London, Arnold, pp. 306–16.

Davis, S.T. and Sheely-Adolphson, P. (1997) Psychosocial interventions. Pharmacological and psychological modalities. *Nursing Clinics of North America*, **32**(2): 331–42.

Gorman, K. (1999) Sickle cell disease. *American Journal of Nursing*, **99**(3): 38–43.

Judkins, K. (1998) Pain management in the burned patient. *Pain Reviews*, **5**: 133–46.

Kleinman, A.R. (1988) *The Illness Narratives: Suffering, Healing and the Human Condition*, Basic Books, New York.

Levi, R., Hulting, C., Nash, M.S. and Seiger, A. (1995) The Stockholm spinal cord injury study Part I – Medical problems in a regional SCI population. *Paraplegia*, **33**: 308–15.

Lewindon, P.J., Harkness, L. and Lewindon, N. (1998) Randomised controlled trial of sucrose by mouth for the relief of infant crying after immunisation. *Archives of Disease in Childhood*, **78**: 453–6.

McCaffery, M. and Beebe, A. (1994) *Pain: Clinical Manual for Nursing Practice*, London, C.V. Mosby.

Madjar, I. (1998) *Giving Comfort and Inflicting Pain*. Alberta, Qual Institute Press.

Maue, F.R. (1986) Functional somatic disorders. Key diagnostic features. *Postgraduate Medicine*, **79**(2): 201–10.

Merskey, H. and Chandarana, P. (1992) Chronic pain problems and psychiatry. In Tyrer, S. (ed.) *Psychology, Psychiatry and Chronic Pain*, Oxford, Butterworth-Heinemann, pp. 45–56.

Mills, H. and Horne, G. (1986) Whiplash – manmade disease? *New Zealand Medical Journal*, **99**: 373–4.

Modell, B. and Anionwu, E. (1996) Guidelines for screening haemoglobin disorders: service specifications for low and high prevalence. In *Ethnicity and Health: Reviews of Literature and Guidance for Purchasers in the Areas of Cardiovascular Disease, Mental Health and Haemoglobinopathies*, CRD Report 5, University of York, NHS Centre.

Parnell, T.F. and Day, D.O. (eds) (1998) *Munchausen by Proxy Syndrome: Misunderstood Child Abuse*, London, Sage.

Payne, R. (1989) Cited in McCaffery, M. and Vourakis, C. (1992) Assessment and relief of pain in chemically dependent patients. *Orthopaedic Nursing*, **11**(2): 13–27.

Potter, R.G. (1998) The prevention of chronic pain. In Carter, B. (ed.) *Perspectives on Pain: Mapping the Territory*, London, Arnold, pp. 186–94.

Reesor, K.A. and Craig, K.D. (1988) Medically incongruent chronic back pain: physical limitations, suffering and ineffective coping. *Pain*, **32**: 35–45.

Schechter, N.L. (1985) Pain and pain control in children. *Current Problems in Paediatrics*, **15**: 1.

Sheridan, R.L., Petras, L., Lydon, M. and Salvo, P.M. (1997) *Journal of Nursing Care and Rehabilitation*, **18**(2): 139–40.

Siddall, P.J., Taylor, D.A. and Cousins, M.J. (1997) Classification of pain following spinal cord injury. *Spinal Cord*, **35**(2): 69–75.

Skevington, S. (1995) *Psychology of Pain*, Chichester, John Wiley & Sons.

Stimmel, B. (1989) Adequate analgesia in narcotic dependency. In Hill, C.S. Jr and Fields, W.S. (eds) *Advances in Pain Research and Therapy*, New York, Raven Press, pp. 131–8.

Sutherland, S. (1996) Procedural burn pain intensity under conditions of varying physical control by the patient. *Journal of Burn Care and Rehabilitation*, **17**(5): 457–63.

Symonds, T.L., Burton, A.K., Tillotson, K.M. and Main, C.J. (1996) Do attitudes and beliefs influence work loss due to low back trouble? *Occupational Medicine*, **46**(1): 25–32.

Thomas, V.J. and Westerdale, N. (1997) Sickle cell disease. *Nursing Standard*, **11**(25): 40–7.

Thomas, V.N. (1998) Sickle cell disease pain. In Thomas, V.N. (ed.) *Pain: Its Nature and Management*, London, Baillière Tindall, pp. 176–93.

Thomas, V.N., Wilson-Barnett, J. and Goodhart, F. (1998) The role of cognitive-behavioural therapy in the management of pain in patients with sickle cell disease. *Journal of Advanced Nursing*, **27**: 1002–9.

Turner, J.A. and Romano, J.M. (1984) Self-report screening measures for depression in chronic pain. *Journal of Clinical Psychology*, **40**: 909–13.

Tyrer, S.P. (1992) *Psychology, Psychiatry and Chronic Pain*, Oxford, Butterworth-Heinemann.

Ulmer, J.F. (1998) Burn pain management: a guideline-based approach. *Journal of Burn Care and Rehabilitation*, **19**(2): 151–9.

Wagner Anke, A.G., Stenehjem, A.E. and Stanghelle, J.K. (1995) Pain and life quality within two years of spinal cord injury. *Paraplegia*, **33**: 555–9.

Walding, M. (1991) Pain, anxiety and powerlessness. *Journal of Advanced Nursing*, **16**: 388–97.

Walker, I., Holloway, I. and Sofaer, B. (1999) In the system: the lived experience of chronic back pain from the perspectives of those seeking help from pain clinics. *Pain*, **80**: 621–8.

Walsh, M. (1993) Pain and anxiety in A&E attenders. *Nursing Standard*, **7**: 40–2.

World Health Organization (1986) Cited in McCaffery, M. and Vourakis, C. (1992) Assessment and relief of pain in chemically dependent patients. *Orthopaedic Nursing*, **11**(2): 13–27.

Index

A

A beta fibres 9–12, 21, 94
A delta fibres 6–7
accident and emergency departments 63–4
accountability 121
acupressure 93–4
acupuncture 93
acute pain 4, 12, 18–22, 28, 52–4
acute pain services 54–6
addiction 17, 22–3, 114, 117–18, 170
adjuvant drug therapy 87–91
admission procedures 32
advantages of pain assessment 31–2
affective dimension 29
affective-motivational 18–19
age 36
agonist 16, 29
allodynia 163
amitriptyline 88
anaesthetist 55
analgesics 57–72
antagonist 17, 29
anticonvulsants 88–9
antidepressants 87–8, 163
antihypertensives 89
antispasmodic agents 89
anxiety 20, 90, 98, 160, 166, 167
appendicitis pain 8
aromatherapy 95
around-the-clock dosing 68
arthritis 136–7
aspirin 58
asthma 58

B

baclofen 89
balanced analgesia 67–8

behaviours 137–8
believing pain 85, 110
benzodiazepines 90
bisphosphonates 91
body language 137–8
bone density 82
bradykinin 13–14
brain-injured patients 141
buprenorphine 16, 64
burns 159–62
buscopan 89

C

c fibres 8–9, 21
cancer pain incidence 3
capsaicin 90
carbamazepine 89
catastrophising 178
central control 12
central pain 163
centrally acting drugs 104
cervical sprain syndrome 177
changing dressings 160
changing practice 44–6
chemotherapy 91
CHEOPS assessment tool 145
childbirth in ethnic minorities 149–50
children 37
chronic benign pain 28
chronic malignant pain 28
chronic non-malignant pain 82–3
chronic pain 4, 28, 82–5
chronic pain clinics 102–4
clinical governance 121
clinical nurse specialist 55
clinical psychologist 55
clonidine 89
codeine 59

cognitive aspects 11–12
cognitive dimension 29
cognitive impairment 36–7, 135–40
cognitive-behavioural therapy 104, 165
cognitive-evaluative 18–19
cold therapy 97, 147
colic 62, 89
combination pain scales 40
comfort 75, 147
commonly used analgesia 57
communication 44, 112, 115–17
compensation 177–8
constipation 60, 95
control 38, 97, 160, 178
controlled drugs 121–2
coping strategies 74–6, 82, 86
corticosteroids 104
cost 104, 122
COX-2 66
CRIES assessment tool 143–4
Crown report 123
cultural background 85, 148
cultural beliefs 38
cutaneous stimulation 94–7
cyclo-oxygenase 13

D

definitions of pain 4–5
delta receptor 29, 15–16
denying pain 34
dependence 23–4, 170
depression 167
Descartes 2–3
descriptive scales 40
dextropropoxyphene 60
diabetes 83, 137
diamorphine 61–2
diazepam 90
diclofenac 65
dihydrocodeine 60
disability allowance 176
disfigurement 159
distraction 12, 75, 147, 161
dorsal horn 5, 6, 20, 21

dressing changes 160
dynorphins 14–17

E

education 55, 110–11, 151
elderly 3, 36–7, 134–40
emotion 34
empathy 100, 110
endogenous opioids 14–17
endorphins 14–17
enkephalins 14–17
entonox 66–7
epidural analgesia 71–2
ethnic minorities 148–50
evidence-based practice 52, 104, 119
exercise 101

F

facial expression 34, 137–8, 143–5
family 179
fast pain 6, 16
fatigue 101
fear of addiction 117–18
fear of injectons 117
first pain 6–7

G

gabapentin 89
Gate Control Theory 3–4, 10–12, 17–20
gender 38,
guanethdine 104
guided imagery 98–9

H

health care professionals 35–6, 110–15, 120
heat therapy 96–7
heroin 62, 173, 174
high mental stress 178
how to assess pain 33
hypochondiasis 167–8

I

IASP curriculum 124
iatrogenic consequence 77
ibuprofen 65
implications of the pain 118
improving practice 113–15, 124–5
indomethacin 65
inflicted pain 54, 160
influence of the family 179
information giving 20
initial health assessment 32
insomnia 88
institutional policies 121–2
intermittent pain 28
interprofessional pain education
    123–4
intractable 28
intractable pain and secondary gain
    175–80
intramuscular analgesia 117
ischaemia 83
isolation 100–1, 175

J

journal group 142

K

kappa receptor 15–16, 29
ketamine 90
ketorolac 65

L

lack of accountability 120
lack of knowledge 22, 25, 110–15
laxatives 68
learning disabilities 141
leukotrienes 13–14
limitations of prescribing 123
link nurse 142
litigation 177–8
Liverpool Infant Distress Score 143
locus of control 71, 99
London Hospital Pain Chart 40–1

low back pain 77, 83, 177–8
low expectation about pain relief
    117

M

malingering 175
massage 12, 74, 94–5, 147
maximising analgesia 67–70
mefenamic acid 65
methadone 62
minimising pain 115–16
monoamine oxidase inhibitors 62
mood disorder 166–9
morphine 14, 21, 61
mu receptor 15–16, 29
Munchausen syndrome 168
muscle
    spasm 89
    tension 74
    wasting 82
musculoskeletal pain 90
music therapy 74, 99
myths and misconceptions 17, 22,
    33, 61, 111, 115–16, 141

N

nalbuphine 63–4
naloxone 16–17, 64
naproxen 65
national survey 3
needlestick 146
neonates and preverbal children
    141–8
neural plasticity 18, 21
neurological abnormalities 35
neuropathic pain 89, 163
nitrous oxide 66–7
n-methyl-D-aspartate acid (NMDA)
    21, 90
nociceptors 5–12
non-malignant pain 83
non-pharmacological approaches
    72–6, 92–101

non-steroidal anti-inflammatory drugs 13, 65–6, 104
non-verbal behaviour 137–8
non-verbal communication 34, 137–8
noradrenaline 20
norpethidine 62
numbers needed to treat (NNT) 58, 104
numerical scales 40
nurses response to pain 149

O

oedema 89
opioid receptors 6, 14–16
opioid-induced itch 64
opioids 7, 8, 13–16, 22, 29, 59–64, 91
opium poppy 14, 61
organisational aspects 119

P

p6 point 89
pain
    assessment 8, 31–5, 136–45
    assessment scales 38–44
    behaviour 35, 101, 143–5
    beliefs 3
    chemicals 5, 12, 13–17
    diaries 41, 140
    education 55
    expectations 33, 53
    experience 3–4, 17–18, 36
    expression 41
    in the community 3
    modulation 13–20
    perception 12, 17
    sensation 6–12
    stimulus 2, 13, 18, 20–1
    tolerance 148
Papaver simniferum 14
paracetamol 58
patient barriers to effective pain management 115–18
patient-centred care 116, 119, 121

patient-controlled analgesia (PCA) 70–1
patients' perspective 52–4, 83–5
perioperative care 56
peripheral neuropathy 83
persistent 28
pethidine 62
phantom limb pain 28
pharmacist 55
pharmacological approaches 57–72, 87–91
phenazocine 63
physical dependence 170
physical signs of pain 34–5
physical techniques for managing pain 92–7
physiological response 35
piroxicam 65
platelet adhesiveness 13
pneumothorax 67, 93
poor job satisfaction 178
postoperative nausea and vomiting 94
pre-emptive analgesia 21
premenstrual symptoms 95
presencing 56
primary nursing 121
professional collaboration 102
prostaglandins 13, 65
protocol development 146
psychological dependence 22
psychological interventions 97–9, 104, 161

R

radiotherapy 91
referred pain 28
reflexology 95
regional nerve blocks 91, 104
relaxation 74–5, 97–8, 104, 147
relief from responsibility 178
renal colic 62
renal function 13
respiratory depression 16–17, 23, 111

respiratory function 54
Reye's syndrome 58
rheumatoid arthritis 136

S

sea bands 93–4
second pain 8
secondary hyperalgesia 21
self-esteem 101, 175
sensitisation 13
sensory-discriminative 18–19
serotonin 20
Short-form McGill Pain
    Questionnaire 41–2
sickle-cell disease 164–6
side effects of opioids 16
simple descriptive scales 39–40
skilled companionship 76, 86
social activities 100–1
social policy 176–7
societies expectations 157
somatic 29
somatisation disorder 168
spinal injury 162–4
stereotyping 149–50
steroids 89, 90
sublingual analgesia 117
substance abuse 169–75
substance P 13–14
substantia gelatinosa 8, 12, 18
sucrose 146

T

The Patient's Charter 149
tolerance 23, 170
topical NSAIDs 104

touch 9
tractable 29
transcutaneous electrical nerve
    stimulation (TENS) 73, 95–6,
    104
trigeminal neuralgia 89
trust 110
trusting therapeutic relationship 100

U

UKCC Code of Conduct 92, 120
urinary retention 64

V

vasoconstriction 97
venepuncture 54
verbal communication 33–4
visceral 29
visual analogue scale 39
visual displays of pain 34
vulnerable 131

W

weaker opioids 59–60
when to assess pain 32
why treat acute pain 54
wind up 21
withdrawal 23, 171
work demands 119–20
work-related stress 178
World Health Organization 3, 68